HEALTH
& TRAVEL

HEALTH
& TRAVEL

JOHN CHUN

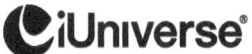

HEALTH & TRAVEL

iUniverse books may be ordered through booksellers or by contacting:

iUniverse
1663 Liberty Drive
Bloomington, IN 47403
www.iuniverse.com
1-800-Authors (1-800-288-4677)

Because of the dynamic nature of the Internet, any web addresses or links contained in this book may have changed since publication and may no longer be valid. The views expressed in this work are solely those of the author and do not necessarily reflect the views of the publisher, and the publisher hereby disclaims any responsibility for them.

Any people depicted in stock imagery provided by Getty Images are models, and such images are being used for illustrative purposes only. Certain stock imagery © Getty Images.

ISBN: 978-1-5320-4268-3 (sc)
ISBN: 978-1-5320-4269-0 (e)

Library of Congress Control Number: 2018902121

Print information available on the last page.

iUniverse rev. date: 03/06/2018

PREFACE

This is a book about how to live healthy and long.

The way to live healthy and long is following 3 things, followed by relatively easier another 3 things.

Altogether 6 things, that I am offering, along with your secret if you have one or more. Out of those 6, some are easy, some are somewhat difficult.

First 3 things are

1. exercise, the most important of all, then 2. drink water wisely, and 3. sleep well.

Then, next 3 are

4. take one baby aspirin in the morning, and 5. take one Zantac at night, and 6. keep oral hygiene good.

It is important to stay healthy untill the time comes when "the One" who sent us here finally calls us to come home, a time for us to "fade away."

Basically, what I'm dealing with in this book is physical health. And, mental health is psychiatrist's, psychologist's, priest's, or preacher's job, not mine.

About 40 years ago, I came to America, the land of opportunity.

40 years later, it is time for me to return the favor to America.

I devoted majority of my life treating sick people, with one ailment or another, sometimes many. Now, I'm going to leave this responsibility to physicians of next generations, who have more knowleges with better idea.

Throughout this book, I'm advocating on unhealthy people to bocme healthy one, and healthy ones remain healthy or healthier.

Contents

CHAPTER I.

HEALTH

We have to be healthy, regardless of age, young or old. But, as we grow older, health becomes more and more important, and the top of the priority of our lives.

When we were young, health was not so important, always at bottom of all the prioties and was one of those things that we took it for granted.

Of course, health becomes more important than money or fame with age. You cannot buy health with money, certainly not with fame.

In this book, I'm going to show exactly how we can live healthy and long, so that my way becomes your way, and then my way and your way become our way. Hopely, with our way, we all live healthy and long.

That is the goal of this book.

So far, I have been busy to help people who are physically sick. My goal was totally to treat the disease.

But, from now on, my goal is going to be different. Maybe entirely opposite. Because I'm treating people, not the disease.

1

I'm going to look for the answer, in search of the solution of this important question," how to live healthy."

Basically, in this book, I'm going to focus on turning the unhealthy healthy, and keeping the healthy healthy or healthier.

When we are talking about healthy living, many people immediately consider something like magic water, or mysterious pill, or strange food, etc.

In reality, many people invest, ie waste lots of money, and precious time just doing exactly what I said above, looking for a magic rather than true solution.

In that regard, we immediately can think of someone whose name is Emperor Quin Shi Huang of ancient China, who beame famous for the persuit of the eternal youth through medicinal herb.

He sent out his generals throughout the country, and when they came back with empty handed, no one survived Emoeror's anger. Through him, we learned valuable lession, that such an effort has its own limit, which is failure and waste.

Unfortunately, recent study showed that our aging process begins at the age of 26.

In other words, ever since we are born, we are marching toward youth, and then at the age of 26, we all stop becoming any younger, instead we all marching toward the opposite direction of what we have been doing ie aging.

We put our first step toward aging, ie degenerative change, at the such a young age of only 26.

As we all know, this degenerative change, ie aging is very much insideous, that the process is so slow and almost invisible.

We may not recognize it untill the ageof 40 or 50.

It showes itself slowly but surely when the time comes.

On the surface, the skin gets wrinkles, the height itself shrinks, on the top of it the spine bends.

It is quite unfair to have changes externally, but there will be universal changes, meaning we age inside as well, which means wherever blood vessels go, our body will undergo degenerative changes.

There is no exception inside out. When we age, we age everywhere.

When those times come, such a illnes like common cold, or flu or simple fatigue and etc, which never bothered us before when we were young, will make certain to make my life miserable.

On the top of that, accumulated stresses throughout our difficult life, in combination with degenerative changes make our lives more difficult.

It used to be non of my concern in the past when I was young. It used to be someone elses' problem.

But, now it is my problem, too.

Anyway, modern science, or advanced moern medicine is absolutely unable to give us any solution to reverse the natural course of degenerative changes.

At least, in our generation, or in the next 10 generations or so, there will be no solution for this delicate mysterious problem. Not even we can see the solution on the horizen.

Probably, no matter how advanced our science might be, this will remain forever unsolved as mystery of human body. We would be better off if there is no answer, no solution for this.

Let's suppose somebody, a crazy scientist found the solution for the aging process, then what happens if all the people of the world know the secret, and remain young without getting old at all?

If only a few of us, or just me only owns the Fountain of Youth, it seems there will be no problem.

But, just imagine how the world looks like if everybody knows the big secret of eternal youth.

As a matter of fact, like the movie produced by Steven Spielberg, "Back to the Future", if we can freely go to the future and the past and come back and forth with a vihecle looks like a automobile, what will happen?

What kind of world we will be living?

Suddenly, if our ancesters of Civil War era show up in front of us with a lot younger looking men or women than me or my children? What kind of family issues do we have to deal with?

The other way around.

If I, myself, show up in front of my great, great, great grandchildrens with younger looks than them, who will be old or young generation of this 'dysfunctional' family? Who will be in charge of my 'reversed(?)' family? Who is senior? Who is junior?

How do we call each other? How do I call my father, whose physical age is much younger, and intelligently much immature than I am, or my son who is older and much more mature than my father.

4

What is going on here?

Or, as another way to solve the problem of aging, like the movie in, "the Curious Case of Benjamin Buttons" starring Brad Pitt, who becomes an ugly old man in the middle of the movie, then suddenly one day, reverses the course of aging, gradually becomes younger and younger, finally becomes a baby at the end of the movie.

So, the best solution for this question, in my opinion, would be we have to turn this unaviodable bad friend, ie aging process into managable living partner of my life and move forward. As we are intellectually becoming old, mature, and wise, we all learn to accept this reality. Getting old has to be a learning process to achieve the ultimate maturity and wisdom of our lives.

As a matter of fact, aging ie degenerative change, ultimately the issue of dying or death, does not have to be our worst enemy or unavoidable curse imposed by the Creator of the Universe, rather, we have to turn what appears to be the Curse of Angry God into Blessing of Loving God.

In that sense, General McArthur's farewell speech makes so much sense to all of us, which is:

"Old soldier never die: just fade away."

Yes, we are. We, all are soldier of life, who "just fade away" at the end,

We are not going to die at the end, we just fade away.

When the curtain comes down, we just fade away slowly and quietly without making any noise.

Simply because I was not the one who made the decision, or the plan to come to this world, that does not mean that I have to die without any consideration of my own decision, but we have the choice to "just fade away" on my own.

We are not a mere presense here on earth and then disappears helplessly, hopelessly at the end. We all choose to fade away when the time comes.

When the stage of my life gradually darkens, and the curtain comes down slowly from the above, accepting that my time finally is here, then we "just fade away" to meet the One who send us this wonderful world.

So, aging itself, further more, the issues of dying or death is not the tyranny of revenging, and/or punishing God, it is that we are in the process of connecting the dots of life, and it is a part of learning process that it is endless, ever lasting love and blessing of Living God.

We need to have the wisdom to make this aging process, ie bad friend to turn into our good friend, ie blessing as we grow older.

So, do not waste your hard earn money and God given precious time chasing after proven lies.

Come along with me to see if you can find a truth or two, so that you find and maintain your health as you grow older.

Here, I'm going to introduce to you several, to be exact 6 of them, that wil show you how to digest the degenerative changes, ie aging, and to live long and healthy untill the time that we "just fade away."

> First, Exercise appropriate for your body
> Second, Drink water wisely
> Third, Sleep well

While harmonizing above 3 things.

Then, I recommend 3 more, 2 of those are easy, but 1 of them might be a bit difficult.

2 easy one first, Which is: take one baby aspirin in the morning, and take one Zantac in the evening or at night. And, the last, but not the least, keep inside of our mouth clean. Although it is not my area of specialty, it's so important.

When I talk about '**Exercise**'

I'm going to discuss about why we have to exercise, which exercise is good, or better than the other, that will give us the best result to our body, how to achieve thr goal.

When I talk about the '**Water**'

I'm going to discuss about what kind of water is good for our body, and how.

When I talk about '**Sleep**'

I'm going to discuss sleep disorder in general, and how to treat the problem of insomnia.

When I talk about '**Aspirin and Zantac**'

I'm going to discuss about the reason why we have to take those medicine.

When I talk about '**Dental Hygiene**'

I'm going to discuss extensively how we can, and what is better, or best way to eliminate gum disease, along with Hallitosis, ie Bad Breath

At the end of each chapter of the above, I always make sure to mention about the solution, the answer, how to solve the problem.

CHAPTER II.

TRAVEL

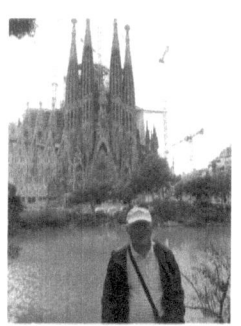

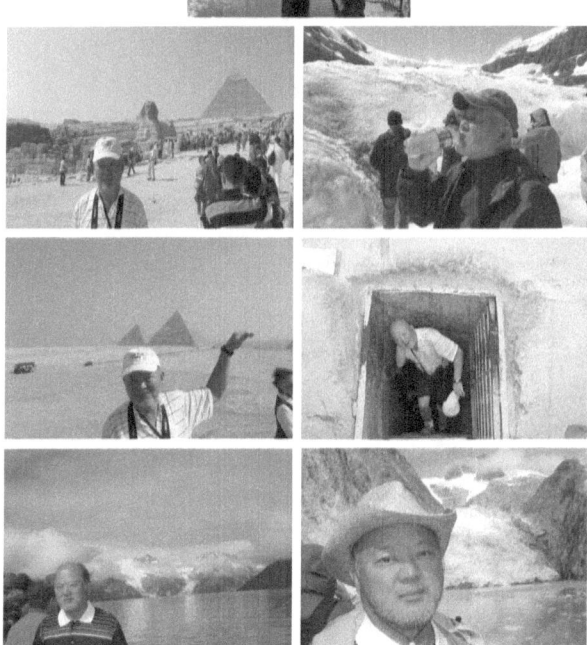

Second to the last of 8 sibling, that's who I was.

Having too many bosses, I always wanted peace and quiet away from the noises and bosses.

In order to find a get-away solution for the peace and quiet of on my own, I chose traveling all by myself, or with a few of my best friends.

I had too many bosses in my early life. I had to find my own freedom in the middle of nowhere, such as at the top of a mountain, or sand dune next to the ocean. I loved the space that a small tent is prividing, only one person or two.

I fell in love with the feeling of the liberty and freedom, at the moment you step out of your house.

But, the farther you are away from home, the closer you feel, and appreciate about everything you have, your home, your parents, your friends, etc. Even though I am far away from home, I feel ever more close to everything that I have.

So, I become a better person to my family, and friends, ultimately to the society and country I belong.

Probably, that might be the reason why I fell in love with traveling deeper and deeper.

When I was growing up, it was "boys never cry" culture. Under any circumstances, no matter how I feel, I should not show my "precious(?)" tears in front of anyone.

But, lately there were several occasions while traveling, I became a little bit emotional, so that I came close to show tears in my eyes.

Once in Egypt, Rome, and Alaska.

I cannot explain why. It is impossible for me to put it in writing. The best way I can suggest, or describe is that you, everyone of you, visit the same places I went, and hopely feel the same.

When you travel, we will have two different feelings about those places you visited during and at the end of the journey.

The first is a place that you want to come back on and on and on, as many times as possible. In those places, you feel like, and always convinced that you will find something new to enlighten your soul, and never fails you to give you something.

In my mind, I have 4 places like that: Rome, Egypt, Alaska, and Barcelona.

The second is a place that is good to visit, but not good enough to make you to want to come back again, and again. Those places are any places other than the above 4.

I'd like to travel alone or only with a few.

There is advantage and disadvantage on both traveling alone or with a few, and in a group. It all depends on how you take the most of the advantege out of both, by doing research, and studying the place where you going. For example, you will learn a lot more about the history, people and culture in such places like Rome and Alaska, if you travel alone or few. And yet, such places like Egypt, and Spain, it would be better travelling in a group with a travel guide. But, it all depends on your personality and inclination.

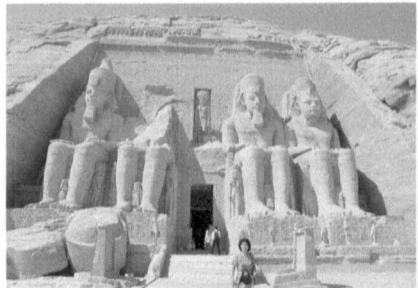 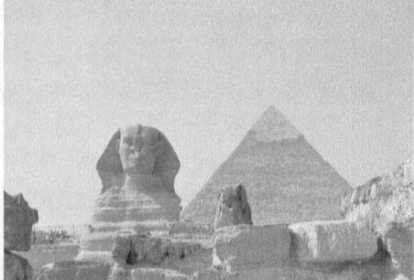

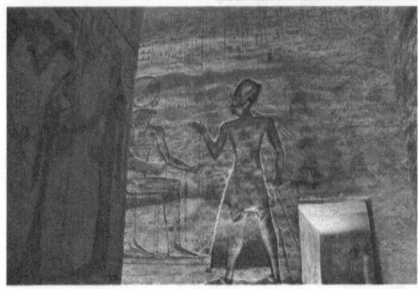

Like anything else in our lives, you have to be healthy first to be able to travel a lot. Work hard, and save enough money, and when you have time to travel, take off, and go where you want to go starting with the place where you wanted to go the most.

You cannot imagine how happy you are, when you are planning and thinking about the travel alone or with a few persons that you know the best.

Just thinking about it, it makes me happy.

Sometimes, when you are travelling, not only you will see places you have never seen before, and meet people you have never met before, but when you are lucky enough, you will taste a food you have never tasted bebore, even though you can eat all kinds of ethnic foods from many different cultures inside America. You, especially your tongue, will remember the taste of some of the food you ate while traveling,

I'm going to give you the lists that are printed in my memory, in my tongue, as well.

Raosted chicken of Lisbon, Portugal

The whole chicken just got out of propane gas grill.

I do not know how it was marinated. But, once I started putting in my mouth, I felt like I was in the heaven.

I like turkey, but never liked chicken in my entire life. I've seen some people who do not like chicken on the table for the same reason just like me.

I grew up in a town where a big market place was located near by my house. I have seen so many chickens being butchered with no mercy at all so many times when I was passing by. I could not eat cooked chicken on the table at home or anywhere else.

I still feel sorry for those chicken who died to please us including myself. I like to eat turkey because I have never seen turkey being butchered. But, I cannot eat chicken because I have PTSD, and I am still going through the childhood trauma. So, I seldom eat chicken, but only fried one, only extracrispy one.

This one, I broke my heart that chickens are tasting this good.

But, it was the best chicken I have ever eaten in my entire life.

Tofu Zigae of Anchorage, Alaska

The soup (Zigae) made with soft tofu, mixed with sea food, and then boiled in a very hot temperature on the top of propane gas flame

You can request to be done mild, moderate, or very hot, I mean spicy hot.

Of course, I always ask very hot.

As you expect, I eat this Korean dish many, many times, and I like it a lot.

Among all of this dish from Korean restraunts in America, and Korea included, this is the best.

There is one Korean restraunt in LA, specializing in this particular dish, which I had several occasion to visit there, it is really good. But, the one in Anchorage is number one on my list.

And, I want to emphasize "taste" is subjective, not objective.

Barbecued Ribs of Yellow Stone National Park

There is a small town, just out side of North Gate of Yellow Stone National Park. I do not remember the name of the town.

At the end of the day, we were looking for a place to have a dinner. We were hungry.

You know better than I do about what is barbecued ribs, how it is cooked. So no need to explain what it is.

We found a restaurant with a small line outside. We immediately knew it's a good one. People who were leaving look so happy. It did not take long to find out how good the food was. Their specialty was barbecued ribs. We all agreed to come back the next day, which we did. It was the best of my list of which is very short.

Everyone of us said that it was the their best.

Sea Food Taco

It happened while at San Juan, Puertorico.

It just happened out of no where. We were walking around the street, and got hungry. Time to have lunch.

We all did not expect that we are going to me the best, not one of the best.

We found a decent reastraunt on a busy street, and ordrered sea food taco with no expectation whatsoever.

To be honest, I ate taco a lot, but no sea food taco, always ground beef taco. I had no sea food taco in my entire life.

It was for the first time, and my last so far. I could not find ant better one.

And, It was the best, still best so far

Water, not food

In Canadian Rocky, there is one place you have a chance to go near the glacier.

Actually you can go on the top of it with the special vehicle you see on Discovery channel and walk around.

There is a small creek, and you can drink the water from it, which I cannot describe how good the taste is. Of course water do not have any particular taste. It is the feeling. I did not want to leave the glacier, but my time was too short. I came down with a bottle of glacier water to my car.

A few hour later, I drank the same water, the feeling was different. You have to drink the glacier water on the top of the glacier, with the same temperature from the creek to have the same feeling that I had on the top of the galcier.

That's why you need to go, and travel the world your way, or my way. No one can do it for you.

I'll talk more about this water, aand other water in the chapter of "Water."

Although it makes me very happy just to talk about it, please remember that I'm not an expert in travelling, not even close.

CHAPTER III.

EXERCISE, THE MOST IMPORTANT OF ALL

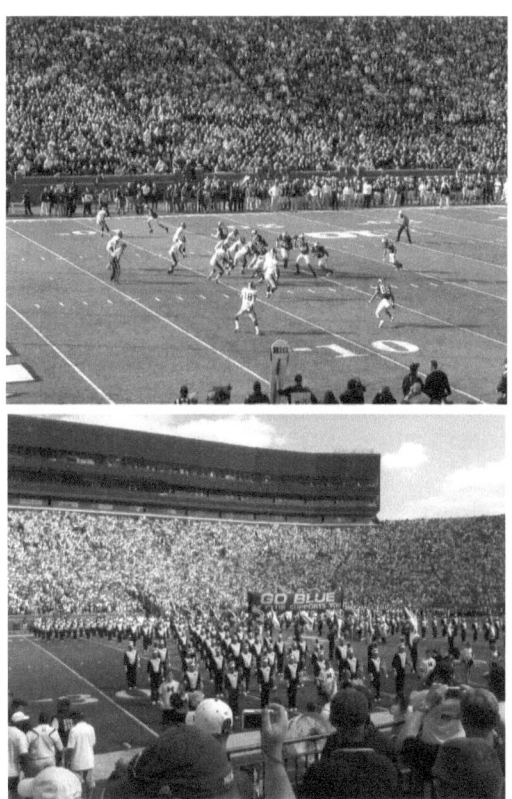

Although there are so many of different and good exercises around us in this world, we have to find the most proper exercise for myself.

As a matter of fact, the main goal of writing this book is to help the readers to find the best exercise that is available and most easily accessible to us while costing minimally.

Then, what kind of changes will the exercise bring to us other than muscle mass increase?

The exercise that I'm about talk is not the kind that only professional asthletes can do, or are doing.

It is about the kind of exercise that anyone, and everyone can do, unless the person is handicapped by either congenital, a condition a person born with, or acquired conditions after birth that keep us from doing it. Othrwise, it has to be we something that we all can do.

Even though we do the same kind of exercise, we can have different results. Even though we do the same kind of exercise, depending on the physical condition of the person, it can be exercise, or the opposite, which is waste of time and money.

Sometimes, even if we use same group of muscle, the result would be different other than exercise, ie called labor.

For one year old baby, walking itself would be vigorous exercise, but for a grown up adult, it is not enough exercise at all. After one hour of walking outside neighborhood, if a health young adult claims that he had a good exercise, there is serious problem.

For a young person with a heart condition, or chronic lung disease walking itself could be a good and vigorous exercise, but for a health young person, it cannot be a good exercise, may be a stress reliever at best.

For an elderly person, walking alone could be a good exercise, but for young and healthy, we only will achieve desired result with vigorous exercise, much more vigorous than walking.

Then what is true exercise?

The answer comes next.

Respiratory Alkalosis

The true face of exercise should be all the muscles involved pushed to the limit, begging to the owner, ie us, being soaked in a profuse sweating, "Please, I cannot go on any longer. I cannot breathe. Please stop." Sweating all over the face and body. This is the way true exercise looks like.

So, when we work out, we have to sweat a lot, have shortness of breath, and lasting at least more than 30 minutes. If the work out is too easy, the effort will be wasted, if it is too vigorous, the chance of getting injury will be high.

This is definition of Exercise, true work out would be;

"For my own health,

-In the process of exercise, all of the muscles involved are exhausted and fatigued out, so -our muscles has to demand much more oxygens than usual, -to meet physiological demand of muscles, our 2 lungs has to function to the limit, as a result, -through the lungs, bring the maximal amount of oxygen into the bioodstream, then into the cells of our body, -at the same time, the carbon dioxide, ie the endproduct of extremely increased metabolism will be pushed out through the lungs.

As result of this high powered gas exchange of the two, uptake of O2 and expulsion of CO2 in the lungs, our body will undergo metabolical transformation from acidic environment (Acidosis) to alkalotc environment (Alkalosis).

Scientifically speaking, we call this phenomenon Respiratory Alkalosis, because alkalosis is caused by respiration, by the lung.

In other words, with true exercise, through respiration, our entire body transforms to alkalotic state from acidotic state.

Respiratory Alkalosis is thr goal of true exercise.

Wait! There is another one.

Endorphin

There is another important element related with true exercise, true work out.

While we are dipping into true exercise, sometimes we get into strange experience, or a feeling like, "What is going on? Or What is happening today?"

Exercise seems so easy today. It has to be hard, and difficult, but, I do not feel tired, or shortness of breath.

As professional athletes often describe, they go into so called "groove"(?). It is hard to describe the feeling. Feel high(?) Have you heard about so called Runner's High(?)

Everything becomes easy. Not tired at all after strenuous work out. We don't have to breathe fast, no shortness of breath, no muscle ache. As a matter of fact, your breathing slows down.

The moment we experience this kind of high(?) feeling, is when our body produces a mysterious substance called Endorphin.

Pituitary gland, located deep inside of our brain, is the one producing Endorphin. That why we feel high.(?)

Actually, we, everyone like you and me, any average person can produce this substance. That precious substance does not belong to professional asthletes only. We all can produce the substance.

When, if we are going through true exercise, true work out, we all produce it, same time when our body transforms from asidosis to alkalosis.

This is the goal of exercise.

Make our body to become alkalotic, and produce Endorphin simultaneously.

Research showed it has similar molecular structure, so named similarly. To emphasize it is produced inside of our body, scientist put Endo- in front of the name,-orphin like morphine which became Endorphin.

This morphine like substance does not cost any money, only requires true exercise, true work out.

When we start producing Endorphin from Pituitary gland, like a person who received small dose of morphine from outside, similar phenomena will occur in our body.

Our heart rate goes down, blood pressure goes down, and breathing goes down. We become very calm. We do not feel much pain when injured due to the anlgesic effect of morphine. Oh no, not morphine, but analgesic effect of Endorphin.

The person feels he moves slowly, but in reality, he is moving very fast, can move as fast as he can, or even faster than ever.

The person even does not feel that much shortness of breath as he should. His heart does not beat as fast as he should, his heart doesn't have to, no need to, even beats slowly, ie bradycardia. As a result, he doesn't get exhausted, instead his opponent gets tired out, and burns out.

So, if I make a formula;

True Exercise = Respiratory Alkalosis + Endorphin

Pistons, Bulls, and Michael Jordan

There are few superheroes in professional sports in our generation. Actually, more than few, but for sure, Michael Jordan is one of them.

He is the living example of Endorphin at work. When we look at him running up and down the basketball court, we are wittnessing Endorphin itself. You see him sweating, but you never see him out of breath, ie short of breath.

Stars of stars are playing against each other at NBA Finals, tied with 3 games each, in the final 7th game, with a few seconds remaining in the 4th quarter, with 2 points behind, and his teammate is inbounding the ball, he picks up the ball, as sonn as he shoots, and the ball leaves his hands, as the game clock expires.

The best defensive player of the opposing team is defending him closely one on one, in addition, and the player on the right and left, 3 out of 5 players of the other team are all over him, and everybody in the stadium literally everybody including people rooting for the home team, and the visiting team, players on the both side of the bench, etc, all stood up jumping up and down, yelling and screaming at top of their voices, the one and only M.J. under the influence of Endorphin, calmy drops 3-point goal, and send everybody home in regulation time, no overtime, shaking everybody's head.

He is the one who always comes to the stadium first, and leave the stadium last. His practice starts bebre the game with other players, but continues after games also. When other players are busy to go home, he remains at the stadium, and continues his routine.

Thus, the Bulls of M.J won the NBA champion titles for 6 times total, 3 times in row, then 1 year off, and another 3 times in a row. He took one year off in the middle because he wanted to be professional baseball player. He tried and failed. What a loser! Then he came back. "And, you know the rest of the story." which will be explained in the chapter of "Rome"

Just a little more about professional bsaketball. To be precise, it is about Detroit Pistons.

Before the heyday of Chicago Bulls of M.J., Detroit Pistons had their own peak, a kind of short(?) one, 2 years in a row of NBA Championship, after losing the NBA Finals to LA Lakers of Magic Johnson, who is the best professional basketball player of all time, in my opinion.

During those 2 or 3 years of Pistons' peak days, Bulls of MJ were no match against Pistons, not even close. Even if he scores more than 50 points, his team still lose to Pistons. Probably, those 3 years of losing badly against the Pistons, MJ must have learned how to lose, and consequently he has mastered how to win.

This is the reason why Pistons had such an 3 excellent years of beating up Bulls and the rest of NBA teams.

First, Pistons had Isiah Thomas, The best shooting guard you will ever see, and Joe Dumas, the most excellent defensive guard, who became the President of Piston's organization, as soon as he retires as a player, who started in one organization and finished his career at the same team, which tells what kind of a person he is, not to mention about as a player.

Isiah Thomas did the same too.

Also, here comes Vinnie Johnson, whose nickname was "Mocrowave" because he was always ready to score a bunch of points immediately he comes in the game.

Second, Then, Centers like Bill Lambeer, of course not only he is tall because he plays center, also he is big, yes he is huge, so that once he takes his position under the basket, no one can push him around. His father was an investment banker, who is the only father who has more money than his son who is current professional basketball player. There is another center, Rick Mahorn. As huge as Bill Lamberr, or maybe bigger. If other player fouls him, other player will fall on the floor. If he fouls other player, the other player will get hurt. Because of these two players, Pistons were called "Bad Boys"

Third, All of a sudden, out of no where, here comes Dennis Rodman. Where did he come from? He started playing regular basketball while in college. His official record tells the story is true.

Fans are even giving him standing ovation if he makes a free throw. Because he rarely makes free throws. But, his rebound, both defenfensive and offensive rebound is outstanding. No player can match him. He jumps higher than anybody else. He jumps so high, opposing centers lose the battle for the rebound. And, he runs faster than anyone else in the court.

So, MJ and Bulls are no match for Pistons at its peak. Joe Dumas covers MJ one on one, then Dennis Rodman gives a hand, then Bulls are no match for Pistons like any other NBA teams.

But, all of a sudden, Rodman moves to Chicago, and "You know the rest of the story."

By the way, few weeks ago, on a TV interview, former Pistons' teammates said Pistons were not the same team after Rick Mahorn was transferred to an expansion team from Minnesotta.

They said Pistons were like old tiger with no teeth. No teams were afraid of Pistons as they did in the past anymore.

Adrenalin

Many people mix up exercise and labor.

Just because you move same group of muscles, if you believe it brings same kind of results, then, it will be abig misunderstanding.

Under certain circumstances, such as to bring foods to the table, or to make more money out of greed, if if it is not for your own health and well being, it is extremely difficult, or almost impossible to initiate to bring Respiratory Alkalosis along with Endorphin.

For example, some kind of physical activities that a construction worker has to go through day after day, it is highly unlikely that his physical activities will give his body Reapiratory Alkalosis, and subsequently Endorphin. His body almost certainly will produce exactly opposite substsnce called Adrenalin.

In these cercumstances, it would be better description to say labor rather than Exercise.

As you can imagine, there would be entirely opposite reaction to our body when our body produces Adrenalin from Adrenal glands located on the top of each of our kidney, compared to Endorphin from Pituitary gland deep inside of our brain.

When Adrenalin is circulating our body, our blood pressure goes up, heart beats faster, breathing unnecessarily faster, our mind becomes anxious instead of calming down.

Of course, there would be difference between a person who reains in the cubicle all day long while struggling with his computer, and a person who works all day outside lifting up and down heavy machinery.

Although there is a significant difference in the amount of muscle activity between the two person, the motivation, and outcome would be entirely different compared to a person who exercises for his or her own health.

So, When a construction worker goes to work in the morning, he says to his wife, "I'm going to work,", never saying, "I'm going exercise." Because, the mind set of "going" out to work for money is entirely different from going out for for true exercise.

Similarly, the other example, Someone, who goes out for golfing, arriving at golf course just few minutes before the tee time. Upon arrival, without having time to loosen up the muscles, at the first tee, he hit the ball in a hurry. Then, instead of walking, comfortabally riding powered cart either gasoline or electric, looking for his ball, and park his cart right behind his ball, and then hit the ball again, and repeating this activities(?), finishes 18 holes.

And then, he says to himself, "I had good work out today."

Everybody can see a problem here. A big problem. After wasting his time and money, if the person says, "I did good." What good did he do?

It makes more sense if he felt s lot of stress got released. In here, do we notice no Respiratory Alkalosis, no Endorphin for sure?

Another worse example.

Combining exercise and stress release, someone who comes to the golf course, he goes home not only without exercise, but also with more stress than before he came. On the green grasses of the field, with cool fresh air, and under crystal clear blue sky, we see some people put more stress on themselves with angry face while betting money, or arguing whether someone violated PGA golf rules, or cheated or not. We, also, see someone chain smoking in between the golf shots.

Definitely, I'm not emphasizing golf itself is bad. It could be an excellent true exercise depending on how you play.

Again, through the true exercise, if we move, or transform our body from acidosis toward alkslosis, the metabolic syndrome of modern era, such as hypertension, type II diabetes, high LDL-cholesterol, low HDL- cholesterol(good cholesterol), and abdominal obesity even coronary artery disease, heart attack and stroke etc that we want to avoid at all cost, will move away, disappear from us, because they cannot survive alkalotic environment of our body along with Endorphin produced by true exercise, and we will be able to live long and health as we want.

Even, cancer says good bye, and leave us.

Just recently, worldly renouned Oncologist, specialists for cancers, agreed and annonced that cancer cells prefer acidic environment rather than alkalotic environment.

In other words, Cancer likes, and loves acidosis. Cancer hates alkalosis. In acidosis, cancer thrives in our body. In alkalosis, cancer cannot survive in our body. They leave our body, or die.

We have to eliminate the matabolic syndrome listed above, as a result of enormous stress and acidosis that we created, which invaded our body being unrecognized by you and me.

But, through good exercise, we give frequent, and numerous chance to our body to become alkalotic environment along with Endorphin, as a result give our body good strength to fight off, and eliminate all those metabolic syndrome, as well as cancers.

That is the goal of this book, my book.

Lastly, there is another medical condition other than Metabolic syndrome and Cancers, that likes acidosis is worse than Metabolic syndrome and cancer, worst of all.

That is a condition that happens to everybody just before dying or death. When we die, we all die a condition called metabolic acidosis, along with respiratory acidosis. That's the end of it.

Next, the good news.

I'mgoing to introduce to you the best "True Exercise" among many of them, in my opinion.

The better news is it does not cost you much.

True Exercise, ie Good Work Out

Let's go and find the best work out for you and me.

Let me begin with conclusion first.

The best exercise to maintain and improve our basic health is exercise of lower extremities. Of course, exercise of upper extremities, chest, abdomen, and waist are important, but exercise of calf muscle should be the most important.

Some people say calf muscle is the heart that located outside, that we can see outside.

This means that if and when our calf is strong, our heart is strong.

With exercise, when and if you make your calf strong, your heart will become strong. Does it make sense??!!

You can catch 2 birds with one stone. This is exactly what you are doing when you exercse your calf muscle. Maybe more than 2 birds, no 3,4,5 and more. I'll explain later.

If I claim that I can catch more than 10 birds with one stone only, not many people would believe me.

But, I do not mind whether people believe me or not, when I tell the truth. As long as I'm telling the truth.

But, one thing bothers me. It's bird. What are the birds going to say? How the birds going to say, if a person says he can catch, or kill 14 birds with one stone?

This is why. And it is true.

1. & 2. As I mentioned above, with exercise of lower extremities, calf muscle gets strong, then our heart gets strong.

3. Our lungs get stronger, too. All the indies of lung function improve with exercise. With exercise, the reason we get shortness of breath is not because we have a problem, or weakness in the lungs, but it is the evidence that our lungs gets stronger, and with shortness of breath, ie hyperventillation, we are developing Reapiratory Alkalosis.

4. With exercise, blood vessels, especially arteries while repeating constrictions and relaxations, becomes more flexible, thus blood Pressure goes down.

5. With exercise, we increase carbohydrate metabolism. As a result, blood sugar drops down.

The best way to decrease blood glucose, and the best way to control sugar problem, ie Diabetes Mellitus. It is better than diet, or pills, or injections, etc. If you combine exercise with diet and drug therapy, the success rate of sugar control will be sky high. If you don't, the failure rate will go sky high

No need to explain more.

6. As mentioned above, blood vessels, especially arteries become more flexible, the incidence of heart attacks and stroke goes low, significantly low.

7. I already mentioned cancer also does not like, actually hates Alkalotic environment. I'd like to say that Respiratory Aikalosis pushes out cancer, or kills cancer. This is not what I want to say, but Oncologists are already saying it.

8. With exercise, in the blood, bad cholesterol(LDL-cholesterol) goes down, and good cholesterol(HDL-cholesterol) will go up. What a miracle!!!

9. If and when we have strong thigh, our back gets strong, too. The back pain leaves me, and my old back comes back.

10. If you exercise lower extremity, not only the muscles become stronger, but also very important joints, such as ankles, knees, and hip joints become stronger.

11. When you exercise well, you sleep well, too. I'll comment more about this in the chapter of 'sleep'. Insomnia goes away.

12. If you work out, you will lose weight. I'll comment more about how to lose weight in the chapter of "How to lose weight" Also, I'm going to mention about interrelationship between fat cell, muscle cell, and Exercise in the same chapter.

13.If you work out, you will not find the word 'indigestion" in your dictionary. No need to explain.

14. As you get older, constipation is one of the many you will end up getting, which you never had when you were young. Because you are not as active as when you were young. Activity or exercise is the key ti avoid this kind of constipation rather than Stool Softner. Get up, and walk around, and work out, instead of taking Stool Softner.

There are few more, but I have to cut it short. Because it is getting too long.

Just one more thing if Ican. Work out is good for ED. That is all. Just ask people who exercise, work out a lot.

All of the above are scientifically proven. I did not make it up. Why should I?

So, the conclusion is exercise, exercise, and exercise.

Now, we are going to search for good exercise.

What would be the definition of "Good Exercise"

First, First of all, it should not cost too much. The cheaper, the better.

If it cost too much, it will be out of the category of good work out such as golf. No matter how good the exercise would be for our body, if it is too expensive to participate, it drops out of the list. Golf itself can be an excellent workout, not only it is too expensive, it consumes too much time, you cannot do it at night, etc and so on.

Second, The result has to be good. The result??? Do you remember Respiratory Alkalosis? And, Endorphin?

Third, It has to be simple and easy to do. It has to be something that you can do under any weather conditions such as raining, windy, snowing, thundering, or lightening, etc. It is something you can do anytime you want even at night.

If it is far away from where you live, such as swimming or tennis court, eyc that it takes too much time to get to there, it drops out of my list.

O.K.

Enough is enough. Let's begin the search!!

Since, I already recommended lower extremity exercise, particularly thigh muscles, We are going to think about following 4 thigh exercises.

1. **Cycling, Biking.**
2. **Jump Rope**
3. **Sit Up**
4. **Stair Exercise, the best of all!**

Before we talk about above 4, let's think about some other excellent exercise such as Tennis and Badminton, jogging, walking, and hiking, etc. These are excellent thigh exercises. No question, but we are looking for the best.

First, Tennis and Badminton.

These are really excellent thigh muscle exercise. Even though it cost a lot to a certain people, compared to the other expensive sports, it is not that expensive.

But, the trouble is you have to go to tennis court to play tennis.

It is one of the best sports to build up stamina, tennacity, etc.

You have one more hurdle to overcome. You have to have one or two good partner. But, he or she is human being, too, who can get sick in bed, or tied up with his or her business, or can go on a vacation like you do.

Because we are all human after all.

And, another problem is, if there is too much discrepancy in ability between the two players. For one player, it is extreme exercise, for the other it is no exercise, not even close.

And, there is one more serious problem.

You can get hurt. Sometimes, you are too slow, or the ball is too fast for you. If you stretch over too much, your ankle, your knee, or your back will inevitably gives out. When you are getting older, healig process slows down. And then if you injure again and again, it will leave permanent damage. Then you have to give up the one you liked, and enjoyed the most.

But, there is few exception. Somebody I know still plays tennis over the age of 70s, and 80s.

So, it is up to you, but not many can do this.

In case of Badminton, ciecumstances are similar.

Next, walking and jogging ie running

These are also excellent exercise. But, if you are doing this outdoor, it has significant limit such as weather and place.

You need to have a good place to run close to you, and if it is raining, snowing, or windy, you cannot go out.

Due to these limitation, if you join a fittness center, you have to go there to do your favorate workout.

1. Cycling, Biking

This is really good exercise. It used to be my favorate one, but I had to give it up. Just thinking about it, I feel like I'm flying. Let me explain you why.

First of all, you need to have a good place to ride bicycle nearby, unless you do it with ststionary bike. Otherwise, even if you have a good equipment, it's no use. You have to go outside.

If weather does not help, you cannot do it, no matter how desperately you want to do.

It is no joke, when you are thinking about the cost. The more it looks good to you, the more it will cost to you like when you are buying a car.

You have to consider the risk of accidents. Because of my mistake as a bike rider, I can hurt myself, or others if you are not focused.

By the same token, I can get hurt seriously by other's mistake.

You need to have certain level of skills or talents to fix it, when your equipment breaks down.

This was the part of the reason why I had to give up cycling, because I have congenital deficiency in fixing anything.

If you choose indoor bike, you can eliminate many of the above limitation, but you have to make a small sacrifice, small space of your house, or your apartment.

2. Sit-up

There is no limitations. No ploblem with expenses, no cost for this exercise. you can do anywhere, no problem with weather at all.

So many of advantages compared to othes, but the one and only diadvantage is that it is monotonous. It is so boring.

But, if you do this exercise properly, you will have enormous result. You are going to see enormously strong thigh muscles, which reflects that you have a strong heart.

But, it is not a good exercise as a primary tool, although it is good exercise as secondary tool.

3. Jump Rope

Another excellent exercise!

I recommend this exercise to as many people as possible combining with other exercises.

It is so easy and simple, but the result is impossible to describe.

You can do anywhere. You can do this under any kind of weather.

I recommend this exercise highly, but as secondary tool.

With one warning. Because there are some people who cannot, or should not do this exercise. Someone, who has back problem, should not do this exercise, especially in the lumbar spine area.

Our spine has gentle S-curve, to protect our brain, minimizing the Impact coming from below. So, lumbar spine is the one with curve to protect our brain.

Then, who is, or what is protecting our lumbar spine. No one. There is no mechanism protecting lumbar spine.

When we jump up and down, our lumbar spine receives more than 90% of the impact coming from below.

This is the reson why.

If you have low back problem, don't do this exercise.

4. Stair Exercise

This the best exercise of all, in my opinion, hopefully it is going to be your best, too.

Quickly, let's go over a little disadvantage. You have live either in high-rise apartment building or near one of those.

But, if you live in a high rise apartment, or at least taller than 5 story apartment, or you are living next to a tall building readily accessible, this disadvantage quickly disapprers.

And, there is one small caution.

Do not run up and down. You have to do it slow. You do not need to do it fast.

Surprisingly, it is more effective if you do it slow. If you do it fast, only the risk of accidents would go up.

To a person who had bad experience of fall in the floor of a swimming pool, or in a sauna, no need to explain.

Particularly, if you are a person who has ankle problem, knee problem, hip problem, or back problem, do it slow, then increase intensity gradually.

It has nothing to do with exercise itself, but it is good to carry your i-phone while you are doing this exercise.

First, there is a stop watch in the i-phone, so that you can check your performance.

Second, This is more important. In case of accident, you can call someone or 911 for help.

This is a true episode about 911.

It happened to a family who just moved to the neighborhood of Bloomfield Hills from Korea, not too long ago.

It was on one December evening, when they came bak from Christmas shopping. It was cold and windy night. The husband parked his car in the garrage, and closed the door, and started unloading the car. First, he put his children in the bed, then shopping bags.

But, one by one including his wife started passing out. And the husband was also started to lose his consciousness.

He realized that it wae carbon monoxide poisoning, as he remembered that he did not turn off his car's engine. This was his first mistake.

His second mistake was when he went to the phone, he was dialing 119 instead of 911.

At that time, i-phone was still not in the market.

In korea, Emergency call is DIAL-119.

Barely, he remembered it's 911 in America. Finally, he managed to dial 911, then passed out also.

It did not end with no tragedy. Because the police responded real quick, and no one died. But, briefly the husband was under the suspicion of 3 first degre murder by the police.

Why did he dial 119 rather than 911? Is there any reason behind? Untill, they found out that emergency number in Korea is 119.

Now, let's talk about advantages. There are so many.

First of all, the cost. You need to buy a comfortable shoes and outfit. That's all you need, and all you have to do is just go out.

Second, since the stairs are located inside the building, it is not affected by any kind of bad weather, such as rain, snow, wind, storm, etc. Weather does not affect you whether you can do it or not.

You can do it even after the sun went down.

Third, as long as you are not the one who initiated the accident, you are free from any accident. You will rarely become a victim of a accident. As log as you do it slow, and and careful, the chance of accident would be very low.

Fourth, if you live in an apartment taller than 5 floor, where you are going to exercise is in your building. The moment you step out of your door, you can start your workout almost immediately. It is very convinient to do it. You just open the door, and thay's already the start of your exercise.

Why 5 floor? The answer comes very soon.

How to do it, how I did it.

Once, a famous expert in health issues advised in an article on a news paper that it would be very good workout if we would go up and down 10 floors twice at a time. I forgot how often he said we should do.

So, I followed his recommendation, tried exactly the way he said.

I failed. I was so disappointed that I failed. It was too hard. I could not finish.

I overestimated my ability and could not believe that I was such a loser. I failed after a few trial.

I did not realize that I had to start from the bottom to climb up to the top of the mountain.

So, I started from the bottom, not knowing how high the top of the mountain would be.

I changed the format entirely.

I went up and down 3 floors twice at a time. A lot less than what the expert was recommending. It was managible. Never run up and run down.

And, then 3 floors 3 times at a time. Again it was managible, and continued for a while.

Then, little by little, I increased the intensity filled with confidence thay I can do it.

I do not remember in small details. I do not remember how long I did. But, it became 4 floors, 3 times, followed by 4 floors, 4 times. Then, 5 floors, 4 times. Then,5 floors, 5 times.

6 floors, 5 times. 6 floors, 6 times. 7 floors, 6 times.

7 floors, 7 times. And, 8 floors, 7 times then, I could not move up more than 9 floors.

As a matter of fact, I had to cut down. to 5 floors gradually, but went up to 10 times.

So, I do it now 5 floors 10 times ups and downs at a time.

How many times a week? It is a bit simple.

It started twice a week initially. Then 3 times a week and 4 times a week. Sometimes, more than 4 times a week, almost every day, when I feel better.

Then, now it became 3 times a week, it is like every other day. Never go up, or down. It is never like Monday, Tuesday, Wednesday, or Thursda, Friday, Saturday. It is always like Monday, Wednesday, Friday, or Tuesday, Thursday, Saturday.

Now, my routine is 5 floors, 10 times at a time, 3 times a week, only a little bit of variation, rarely goes out of norm.

And, it takes about 40 minutes to complete. 40 minutes of excellent workout.

A small piece of advice to those people who are physically handicapped who cannot do Stair Exercise.

Even though it might take more time and costing a bit more money, I recommend swimming. Go to swimming pool. Actually swimming is the most ideal exercise of all.

We all came out of water, we ought to go to the water.

Exactly speaking, our body consists of 2/3 of water, and 1/3 of soil, meaning 1/3 will go back to soil, 2/3 will go back to water.

Acoording to the Bible, "Men are from dust, so go back to dust." would be 1/3 correct statement, but 2/3 incorrect, because our body is 2/3 of water.

Before we all were born, we stayed in the mothers' swimming pool for over 9 months, and were pushed out of the best environment without my or our opinion being considered at all. 100% not my decision, 0% my decision.

We all did not come out of the most ideal environment. As a matter of fact, we all wanted to stay inside.

Anyway, if we go to the sea or river, and jump into the water, we feel like we came home.

Exercise in the water is the most ideal and the most effective environment. The best physical therapt of all will be the therapy done in the water, and utilizing the gentle resistance of the water.

We all came from the water, so we all go back to the water. We go to the swimming pool filled with water.

So, when we are done here, and when the moment comes for us just fade away, we all go back to the water.

As a result, my water meets your water, then it becomes our water. And, our water meets another our water, then becomes a big river and the ocean in between the big continents.

And, eventually we all meet each other in the middle of the Pacific oscean.

By the way, from time to time, when I'm in the middle of strenuous exercise, I experience strange thing. Sometimes, I do not feel tired, I do not get shortness of breath, I feel very calm. What is it? Can I say it Endorphin ?

I'm going to leave the answer up to you.

CHAPTER IV.

ROME

I recommend a trip to Europe as many times you can.

But, if you are a person tend to focus on one thing, or one place, I recommend Rome, Italy.

There is old saying, "dig one hole, then you will get a good well that gives you excellent water."

As I recommend in the chapter "Travel", you go to Europe in a group setting, visit as many places as you can, then concentrate on one place, and go deeper and deeper that you like.

Rome is the kind of place the more you visit, the more you will want to visit and see that you have never seen before.

Some people, who went to Rome as part of a package tour of European countries, come back and say, "I went to Rome. I have seen Rome." after spending 2 or 3 days only in Rome.

In the old days, wise man asks, "What have you seen in the mountain, while on a speeding horse?"

It is like, after passing through New York in a speeding race car, claiming "I have seen New York."

After just licking outside of a water melon, what if someone says," this water melon is so sweet." What are you going to say to this person.

There are some, but not many, people who travel every coner of the world on foot with a minimum cost of money. They work hard, save enough money, then take off. Of course, they study hard about all those places they are planning to visit, geography, history, culture, etc.

This is what, so called, "travel professionals" are doing. However, majority of us are not travel pro.

So, I suggest to the majority including myself that what most of the people have done so far.

Set the goal, then work hard, and save money. And, when you think that the time has come, take an action.

There are millions different way of travel packages that are available to us.

Take advantage of one of those, once, twice, then become an expert as far as Rome is concerned.

Terminale

I got the impression that it seems like the public transportation of Rome are made not only for the convenience of the citizens of Rome, but also for the visitors, travellors like us.

"All roads lead to Rome"

This was true several thousands years ago in old Roman Empire, and also is true at present time in Rome.

You can go anywhere from the terminale, and come back to the terminal from anywhere.

Terminale is the center of all transportation in Rome.

In Rome, there is only two directions where the public transportation is heading, one is to your destination, and the other is always to the terminale.

After your day's schedule, for whatever the reason is, if you choose to take a taxi, you just tell the taxi driver "Terminale!", then he will take you to the familiar place.

If you buy tickets for public transportation, you can use it everywhere, and anywhere.

The price of the ticket is reasonablly cheap, and of course you can buy certain amount of tickets at a time, so that you do not have to buy every morning. You can carry enough tickets for the day.

You do not have to worry if you run out of tickets before the day is over.

The trick is simple. You can ride the bus without tickets. The mission of public transportation of Rome is for the safety and convinience of the passengers, not money. The bus drive never looks back. He only looks to the front for the safety of fellow human being, citizen of Rome, and equally as important, visitors like me, the driver never looks back to check whether the passengers are putting the tickets in the box. I'm not encouraging you to take free rides, but when you have no choice, you have to do what you have to.

Personally, I'd like to recommend to ride a bus because you can see outside what is going on. Subway train is convenient and fast to get one place to another.

So, when you visit Rome, it is very convenient if you choose a place to stay close to the terminale in a walking diatance, within 10 minutes or so.

When you finished your daily schedule, take a bus or a subway train, always you will end up at a familiar place, then just take a walk.

You can find a good restraunt for dinner, also can have a nice looking bottle of wine, sitting in what it looks like a party store in America.

So, you start your day from the terminale, and finish your day around the terminale.

If you do this as daily routine for a few days, you will already find yourself feeling like you are at home.

Pick Pockets

In Rome, if you carry cash or jewelries in your pockets, it is no longer yours.

As a traveller, all you need to carry in your pocket is small amount of money enough for your lunch, and snacks in case you get hungry or thirsty before lunch or before coming back for dinner. You should not carry all of your money with you for the entire travel. Always keep all the spending money at the hotel's safe, and you carry only money enough for the day. All the money you need for one day is for lunch, snack, and drink like water or pop.

This is not a good subject to talk about, but you have to be careful if there is a risk to lose your money to continue and finish your pleasnt trip untill you come home.

But, it is not suprising to see some kind of fall out, or nagavity, for most of the European countries are the recipient of enormous number of visitors each year, especially during the peak season of travelling.

Most of European countries are very safe to travel, safer than you think. In general, the countries with large number of visitors, the crime rate is low, particularly, crime against travellers is low.

Another warning or advice if you are planning to visit any foreign country, would be "do not go out for shopping", do not waste your time buying things that you can buy here in America.

Sometimes, you are sure that you bought something in the countries such as "made in Italy" in Rome, or" made in France" in Paris, or "made in Briton," in London etc, you will be suprized to find the goods made in different country.

Items are made in the different countryies where the minimum wages are very low. You saw the label with your own eyes when you bought. But, when you come back to Hotel, and look again, the label turned into different countries.

I call this "Magic" but, don't be fooled by this "Magiic"

History of Roman Empire

This is what I do when I go to Italy, specifically Rome.

You have to spend at least a day or two to see St. Peter's Cathedral and Cistine Chapel, and then divide Rome

4 quardrant, spend at least one or two days on each quardrant.

And, if you visit one or two places about one hour or two away from Rome, 7 to 10 days would be enough.

Unlike travel professionals, amateur like you or me will get homesick when we stay away from home more than 10 days or 2 weeks. By then, we are going to miss the comfortable bed of mine we have at home.

Again, once is not enough. I do not know how many times is sufficient the place like Rome. That is why, each time you go and see Rome, you say, "I'll be back."

Like anywhere else, if you want see a place the way it is, you have to study and know the history of the place where you are going to visit. This is particularly true when you go to Rome.

I learn the history of Italy and Roman Empire a bit when I was in high school in world history class. But, that is not enough. Not enough to know the interesting part. We need to know a bit of the behind story. Then, the travelling is going to become to a level of entertainment.

We cannot say, "vini, vidi, vici"("I came, I saw, and I conquered") wherever we go, and came back.

As you can imagine, there is big difference between a person travelling with the significant knowlege of history of the area, and someone who does not. The person with knowledge will come back home with much more konwlege about the place than ever before.

One person might say," I came, I saw, and took pictures."

But, the other person will say, "I came, I saw, and I learned."

After travelling, one person remains the same, or worse because he or she got older, and another person becomes more mature, wiser, and more knowlegible than before, even though this person got older, too. This is the difference.

A bit of history of Roman Empire.

In the beginning, Roma was founded BC 753. Two countries, ruled by the twin brothers, Romulus and Remus, were united by Romulus. Still, it was a small country that no one or countries paid any attention to.

At that time, Egypt was going downhill, but as a country they were still powerful, Greece was becoming a powerful country both militarily and intellectually.

And, right above, on the north of Rome, there was Etruria, a country strong in military, and very skillful people, who can build good bridges, and road.

Down below, on the south, there were many cities run by Greeks, who were good at trade by the sea.

Now, the most scary one, Cartago, a strong and rich country in northern Africa in the area of present Libia, was always ready to invade Italian penninsula. Many times, they come and occupy Sicily, then invade different parts of mainland Italy.

Roma was located in the mid portion of Italian pennisula on the Mediteranian side.

Romans were surrounded by strong enemies everywhere near and far.

But, sooner or later, Romans are becoming stronger by concurring or obsorbing villages, and small countries one by one, and build up the strength.

They become even stronger by implementing the most successful immigration policy in the history of mankind.

When Romans are engaged in a war, and win. Then, the prisoners were given two choices by the commanding general, one is immediate execution or sold as slave, and the other is Roman citizenship. Depending on the circumstances, it is the commanding general who decide the fate of the prisoners whether to execute all of the captured. The worst case of execution by the Romans against any enemy is destruction of everything and everyone.

Once the commanding general decides total destruction, then nothing survives.

One example, and the worst is when they won the war against Cartago, they killed every living things inside, human, men and women, young and old, even babies, animals, and destroy everything standing staright to the ground, then burn everything. In the end, dump salt everywhere so that nothing can ever grow out of the ground.

That is the reason why Jesus was weeping out loud even though all of his desciples were watching and listening, while he was looking at Jerusalem, the Holy Temple, before he died. Apparently he knew what was going to happen to the Holy Temple by the Roman Emperial Army in the near future.

Jesus knew about 50 some years later Holy Temple will be destroyed and demolished by Romans as it happened to Cartago. According to the record, there were a lot of people that came from other countries far and near for the Passover.

After the standoff, almost 600 thousnd people died and 90 thousand captured, and sold as slaves, then the total, complete destruction of thr Holy Temple and the city of Jerusalem.

Among the dead, many of them died of starvation, or communicable diseasees due to shortage of food, and total lack of hygiene because the standoff lasted more than 5 months.

It is not surprizing for Jesus, who knows how much his people were going to suffer, to cry out in spite of his desciples, and his followers were watching him on his side or behind him. He could not control his emotion at all, for only he knew what exactly was going to happen to his people and the Temple.

Why Jews and Romans hated each other that much?

Of course, Romans were the conquerers, and Jews were the occupied. So, it is quite natural that the occupied hate the conquerer. But, why Romans hated the Jews?

Let's consider some other potential factors other than the have and the have not.

Yes, Romans had everything, and Jews had nothing.

But, the Romans know very well that Jews are not paying, or refusing to pay taxes to Roman Empire. Instead, they sent their money to Jerusalem, the Holy Temple.

And, the Jews refused to serve mandatory military service that every citizen of the Roman Empire are proud to serve in the mliltary.

Lastly, at that time, Jews, especially in Rome, are kown to get together every night at a secret place and pray to their God asking his Son to come back ASAP.

His son, Jesus, told his deciples that he will die in a cross, but will rise from the dead in 3 days, and then go to Heaven to see his Father, then he will be back soon.

He never told anyone exactly how soon. So, one of his deciple asked him exactly when he wil be back. His answer was "I do not know. No one knows. Only my father knows."

Because of this ambiguous answer, his people took it the way they want to hear. Certainly they thought he will be back soon, soon enough that they are still alive in this world. The desperate Jews were asking God to send his son back to the world, and build his eternal Kingdom of God. And last, but not the least, to destroy the evil Roman Empire.

We, all, know that he is not here yet, still do not know when. It was their problem then, now it is our problem. Still no one knows when.

Anyway, that was how the Romans punish any enemy of Roman Empire. They demand absolute royalty from the enemy, or else complete wipeout.

When they won the war against Etruria, become even stronger, and strong enough to get the attention of Cartago, especially by Hannibal.

Romans has to go through 2 gruesome, long war against Cartago, especially against Hannibal in second war, the best, the best of the best field general, over 40 years of the first war, and over 20 years of the second war. It took almost 120 long years of struggle, first and second Poeny War.

In the history of mankind, Hannibal is the best of field leader, no one is better than him. Some people say Alexander the Great should be the greatest. To some extent, I agree. But, think about their oponents. Who were their enemies?

Alexander's opponents, enemies were entire world, and everywhere, but they were all amatures.

Hannibal had one opponent, only one enemy, which is the Roman Imperial Army, the war machine, the war professionals, the killing machine.

He almost won the war single-handedly against Roman Emperial Army. What a remarkable achievement.

I do not mind other people's opinion, the difference of opinion. But, in my opinion, Hannibal is the one and only, the best.

After the first Poeny War(BC264-BC241), here comes Hannibal. He inherits his father's will, which is destruction of Roman Empire.

He wanted to attack Romans directly by the sea, but Romans had better, and stronger navy. Romans mobilized every ship they had, so that Hannibal can not land mainland of Italy from the sea.

So, he had to go to Spain first, then to southern France, then cross the Alps then attack nothern Italy.

Victory after victory, he almost took over Rome, but passed by Rome, kept on movig to southern Italy. No one knows why he did not attack the city of Rome,

The second Poeny war (BC219-BC201), also called Hannibal War by the Romans, also ended with Romans victory, Hannibal dies on 183BC,

Cartago disappears from the earth on 146BC and become one of colonies of Roman Empire.

You know the rest of the story.

After the demise of Cartago, Roman Empire becomes even more stronger, bigger and powerful.

They expand, and occupy entire Europe, west of Reine river and northern Africa, part of middle east, and build up the biggest empire in the human history. They become the center of the world. Geographically when we divide Europe, west and east, the benchmark is Rome. When we divide the world west and east, same standard is applied. For example, Asia east, America west. And, middle east is because it is located in between Rome and east.

Like human body gets old with time, Roman Empire gets old, too. They cannot fool the aging. Even the Roman Empire cannot avoid the aging process, ie degenerative change.

But, the everlasting impact of Roman Empire will remain with us, will never go away as long as human history continues.

Although becoming old, and senile, and eventually split into two Empire(?), West and East(396AD). then the West goes down first (476AD), but, the East lasted a thousand more years, and then disappear from the history. (1453AD)

Even after the fall of Roman Empire, the influence, and impact of the Roman Empire continues untill now and maybe forever. Even now, we cannot look at anywhere without seeing their influences such as in politics, military, religion, art, architecture, science, mathematics, diplomacy, immigration policy, sports, transportation, postal service, etc Their influence is everywhere, and ever lasting.

That is the reason why we have to go and see what they have done to our lives, and to my daily life of twenty first century.

Although destroyed, and divided, they led the main stream of Renaissance, and the awakening of Humanity to the level of what we have now.

Especially, in religious world, human became the center of religious belief, rather than the church.

Gradually, but surely, through the teaching of Christ, with the influence of Roman Empire, from the church-centered, and church-oriented religion, human becomes and moves to the center of the religion we have, ie, the Christianity.

The Christianity, that we belive, and I believe, is human-oriented, and human-centered, not church-oriented, or church-centered. Because Jesus told his Disciples and us, that we, the humans, are the most prescious and important creation of his Father, who gave us, the humans, free-will.

It didn't take very long for God to realize that the relationship between Him and human took a nose dive from bad to worse.

No sooner than He realized what was happening, God gave human another thing, something called "responsibility" ie "consequence." When He punished Adam and Eve, He gave specific punishment, ie responsibilities to Man and Woman.

But, if you look at the punishment closely, you will find that He gave the Human profound blessings at the same time. As we grow older, as much as we think we are being punished, we realize that we were given more blessings by Him while we are going through what we think, or appears to be the "punishment(?). It is your homework to figure out what kind of blessings He gave to Adam and Eve, when He kicked out His most precious creation from His home.

So, human was given the "free-will" to do anything or everything, but at the same time, it comes with responsibility, aka consequencies, when human does anything.

Like any other things in our life, we are free to choose the good or the bad with our free-will. When good thing happens after we chose the good, we take all the credit. When bad thing happens after we chose the evil, we take the consequences.

So it is very fair to God, and human as well.

But, there is one thing very interesting; even after we made the bad choice, we are free to think that we chose the good.

Sometimes or many times, even if we commit the sin, we are living, and can live as if we did not commit any sin at all. If we make a bad choice, even though we think we made a good choice, we will end up paying the price of making bad choice.

The result, the consequence, will come to us regardless of what we think, if not sooner, then later. Only God knows exactly when.

This is another advantage of being God. In other words, disadvantage for us. Between God and human, I cannot think of any advantages as human other than free-will, which was given by God in the beginning.

Yes, He is the boss of the entire universe. And, He made us, the humans, to be the boss of this world, and then God is looking at the other side. Yes we, the humans, are in charge of this world.

How good the good God is.

But, there are peoples, countries, or individuals, or religious groups who do not take advantage of or do not make the most out of this God given gift, the free-wills for the good cause of our side or my side.

These group of people or religions are reading their Bible or scripturres, and follow exactly as written. They read and act based on as written. Nothing in betwwen. No free will in between. No interpretaion whatsoever, but read and act.

They do not allow anything comes in between. They think it is insulting their God and their belief if anyone make any attemp to interprete God's intention, to negotiate with God or put free will in between.

Most of the time, they like to read and follow exactly what their founder said, rather than what their founder did, how their founder acted, or even what their founder told them to do. There is no interpretation, no questions, no humanity, no human factor, no free-will to be found in their action.

Jesus showed us the best example of free-will, and how to use it by what he did the night before he was crucified.

He asked not his Father's intention, the reason, or the purpose of what will happen tomorrow. Both knew it so well.

He asked the most desperate request that anyone can ever make with fre will. Of course, I assume he asked his Father the purpose of tomorrow already, but he knew the answer so well, too.

It is no time to ask that question. The time to ask his Father's plan has passed long time ago.

But still, he does his best, and ask his Father make it not to happen what is going to happen the next day. He uses his free-will to the best of his benefit by asking his Father to erase the tomorrw's event from the calender.

But, almost immediately, even before his Father answers to him, he tells his Father to do it as planned.

This is what we have to do with our free-will. Do the best of our benefit by asking God whatever questions we have to our benefits. Who knows if He listens and changes His mind, and does something good for us or for me.

We are free to ask any desperate questions of mine to Father of Jesus Christ, also who is my Father as well.

Most of the times, we know the answer even before we ask like Jesus did 2 thousand years ago.

But, if we do not know, or we were not given the answer, just keep asking the question untill God gives us the answer, or untill he gives up.

Who knows?

Again," how good the good God is" for giving us free-will.

And, for giving us to interpret his intention, and ask for the answer for our own benefits.

While I was studying the history of Roman Empire, my curiosity would take me to the history of Greece, and furthermore to the history of Egypt.

That is why I left my small footprints as much as I can in Abu Simbel in Egypt.

Of course, the founder of Christianity was born in Judea, then the colony of Roman Empire, and to avoid persecution of Roman Empire, he grew up more than few years in Cairo, Egypt. When you go to Cairo, you will visit the village where Jesus grew up with his parents.

After the cruifiction of Jesus, the Christians moved to Rome, the center of the world, and spread the good news like a wild fire from the ghetto of Rome to entire Europe and to the rest of the world with help of the Roman Road, that was constructed by the soldiers of the Roman Emperial Army.

How irony it would be. Roman Empirial Army demolished the Holy Temple of Jerualem. Christianity spreads to the world with help of Roman Road built by the same Roman Emperial Army.

And, "You know the rest of the story."

"Have a Good Day!!!!" by Paul Harvey

Now, he is gone, but there was a famous radio personality in Chicago, whose morning show was heard everywhere in this part of the country. I could hear his unique voice every morning on the way to my work.

His name is Paul Harvey.

At the end of his program, he used to talk about an interesting and unusual story, an incident, an event, or an accident, that happened recently, or long time ago without telling the person's name of his story, then finishes his morning show by spitting out the person's name, and says in his unique way, "You know the rest of the story. This is Paul Harvey. Have a Good Day."

After making his audiences curious the entire time, he finishes the story abruptly. By the time his listners realize what is the true meaning of his stories, he is long gone already.

When you are travelling Europe, or Italy, more specifically Rome, I recommend you to choose the timing during the off-season.

If you travel Rome in peak season, such as in summer time, entire Europe is on vacation, which means it is nightmare for all the travellers.

First of all, avoid the winter season. You have to walk around, sometimes stand outside in a line waiting long time to buy tickets and get in, and so on. It is cold outside. It is not good travelling in winter.

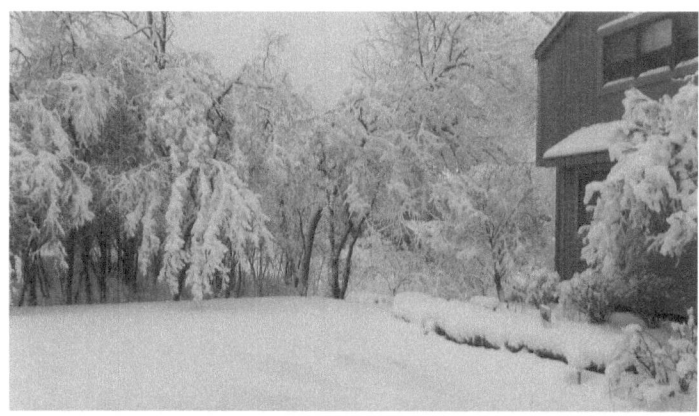

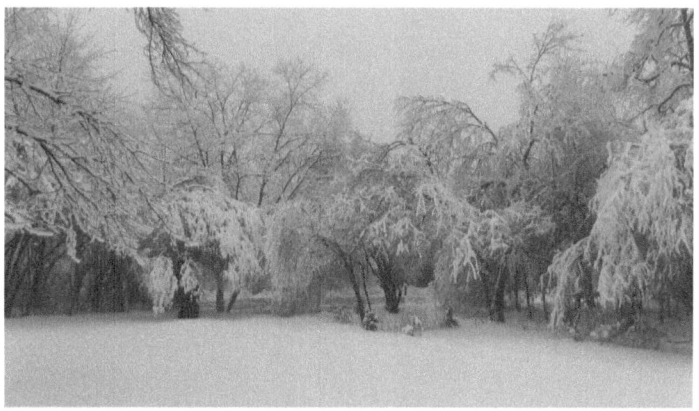

And, during spring break, summer vacation, fall recess, there are too many travellors, you will be waisting most of your valuable time waiting on the line looking at the person's head in front of you, rather than watching famous paintings or sculptures.

So, I recommend the off-season like from mid-Feburuary till mid-March. Again, you have to decide when to travel based on your personal schedule. The period I 'm recommending is still cold, but not winter cold.

It can be cold when the sun goes down, but when the sun is up, and out, it is comfortable outside.

You are going to need the kind of clothes which is very warm and comfortable, light as well. Lightness is very important to minimize the weight you carry.

To satisfy those difficult requirements, I usually go to Costco and do my shopping.

Vatican

Now, we go to Vatican.

It tales approximately 30 to 40 minutes to Vatican if you take a subway at Terminale. So, you start early in the morning.

Then you have to do the thing you do the most when travelling at the entrance; Waiting in line.

There was a long line, we waited about 40 minutes to get the ticket, and went inside. During the peak season, the waiting would be minimally 2 hours according to the tour guide.

When you go inside, go to the Vatican Museum and see the David statue and other famous collections, but do not spare too much time in the museum, because there are whole a lot of things to look that are waiting for you.

Cistine Chapel

It is small chapel attached to St. Peter Cathedral.

It was built as Pope's personal chapel.

But, because of the famous paintings on the ceiling and the walls depicting the Genesis of the Old Testament, it is as famous as, or more famous than any other must-see spot.

Also, this chapel is used when the Cardinals elect new Pope also known as Conclave.

There is a time limit once you get in, you have to come out even though you want to stay a bit longer. You have no choice for other visiters like you.

Also, once you get in you can not take a picture. You have to print in your brain what you see insie.

So, this is one of the places that you have to study or research before you come.

Though you want to stay longer, you have to come out after certain time, your neck will be stiff, because everybody including you has to look at ceiling looking for the painting you want to see, such as the painting that God and Adam trying to reach each other their index fingers are about touch each other like the boy and E.T. in the E.T. movie.

In the movie, E.T touched the boy's bleeding index showing the healing power, but, in the ceiling of Sistine they are not touching with their index fingers, we do not know what is going on here. It's mystery.

According to my friends who went to Cistine Chaple away ahead of me said, they stayed inside as long as they want, and were able to take pictures as many as they want, but the time has changed when I went rhere.

As far as I can remember, Cistine Chapel was closed several times when the new Pope has to be elected, and when restoration work needed to be done, and in progress.

I do not recall the exact year, but it was more than 20 years ago, and closed for several years.

Vatican was having a big headache. Because Cistine Chaple has such a small space, and yet so many people have been in and out so many years. The paintings on the ceiling and wall shows signs of contaminations by human sweats, ferfumes, cigarette smokes, body odor, etc.

Vatican decided to do a major restoration on Cistine Chapel.

Initially, Vatican wanted a group of Italian Exoerts to take care of the restoration, but the expense was so astronomical that they have to look at somewhere else.

When they contacted Japanese Experts, they received an offer that they could not refuse.

Japanese group told Vatican that they will complete the work with no charge at all, but with one condition. The only condition in Japanese plan was nobody can take a photo of Sistine Chapel anymore but themselves.

Vatican gave the permission to take photos only to the designiated group of experts.

The restoration began 1980, and took for 10 years.

Naked God

So, it was a story of restoration that happened in a recent memory.

This story is something that happened at the beginning.

After the wall painting was done, Vatican asked Michelangelo to do the painting of the wall behind thw alter, and the ceiling. He took the job reluctantly because he considered himself a sculpter, not a painter.

While he was painting the ceiling, and the wall behind the alter, he did not allow anyone inside except a few of his apprentices.

But, it did not take too long that the big(?) secret leaked out to the Cardinal who was in charge of the project.

He painted the God naked, without cloths.

Adam can be naked, but it is absolutely unacceptable for God without covering the thing(?) in the middle.

So, the order or the request came from the Carcinal to cover the area(?).

The mission was given to, and accomplished by one of his apprentice, and the Cardinal was given the honor(?) of one of the human's painful face who was sent to hell, and tortured by demons painted by the painter himself, Michelangelo.

If some scientist invent super-eraser, then we might be able to see true(?) God some day.

When we go to the Holy Family Church, in Barcelona, Spain, on the top of one of the entrance, we can see naked Son of God. We have to watch this sculpture with our neck extended like we have to see the ceiling.

The Son on the Cross with arms stretched does not wear clothes, and his VIP (Very Important P?) exposed.

One thing you notice from the many people looking up and watching, is no one, incluing myself, look embarrsed about his "missing" pants.

Historically our ancesters did not wear pants because it was not yet invented, and not available at the time of more than 2000 years ago. Accooding to the bible, before he was crucified, all of his clothes he was wearing was taken away by the Roman soldiers, it is correct historically and artistically that the Son should not wear clothes.

When you are looking at the Son on the Cross who just died, but with the pants on, you might be looking at someone else. And yet, you believe he is the One, you are a true believer.

The Pieta

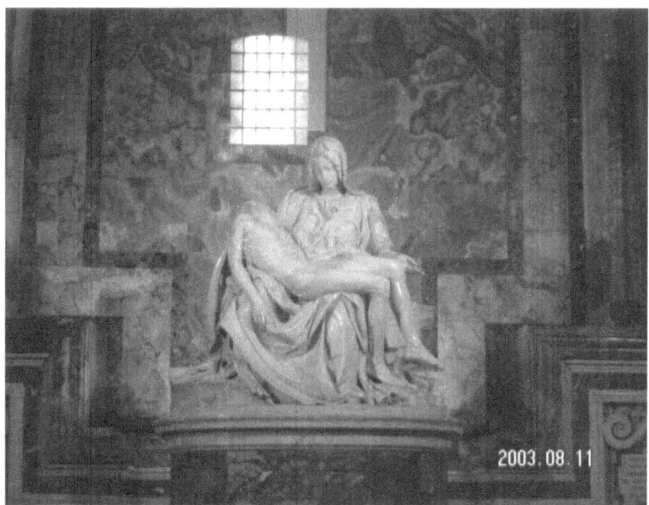

After we were pushed(?) out, or kicked out(?), more politically correctly speaking, told to leave the Sistine Chapel, we go to the top of the St Peters Basilica.

It is not easy to climb up to the top, but you have to do it at least once to look at the entire Vatican City.

Then, come back down, and find a decent restaurant to have a nice lunch.

Finally, we go into St Peter's Basilica. My heart is still racing and pounding due to the electric shock from the ceiling of Sistine Chapel.

There are so many things to see and to talk about inside the Basilica, but I'm going to talk about one thing, only one thing.

I had no idea whatsoever that another, far greater shock that I was about to receive by the same person. Again, my poor soul had no idea what is coming. I was totally unprepared.

Like any other cathedral, we see three big door in the front of the Basilica, the middle door is bigger than the two door on the right, and left.

The door on the right was shut and closed. I noticed the reason why immediately I went inside.

So, I went in the biggest of the three door, then when I turned immediately to the right, my heart frozed. I do not remember how long.

There she was. With her son on her laps.

How many times did I see it in the textbook, magazine, newspapers, and so on.

It is true, and I never realized that it is true that "Seeing is Believing" untill I saw this. You have to see it to convince yourself, and believe what you are seeing.

It is the "Pieta" sculptured by the same person who painted the ceiling of Sistine Chapel.

Everybody's facial expression looks alike. All are hit by a lightening? O No, it is like "Being touched by the gentle hand of the True Love of God," who gave us such a loving mother to us. She is our Mother, and my Mother.

There is an old saying.

"When the husband dies, the wife buries him on the hill." "But, when her child dies, the mother buries the child in her heart."

This is the moment the mother buries her son in her heart.

When we die, no, When we "just fade away", she will do the same for us. When I fade away, she will do the same to me.

Let's not afraid when we die, there is she, who will bury us in her heart like my own mother.

Now, we know that we have 2 amazing ladies, who will willingly give us their warm hearts for me to rest eternally

The entire Christian faith is expressed in this rock. You can feel the entire Bible just by looking at this.

Why waist our time? Just go to Rome, and simply see it. The entire Bible will come to your heart.

This remarkable work was done in 1498, when he was 23, only 23.

When he finished, this young sculptor himself was so glad to see what he did, he could not stay away from it. Every afternoon, or evening at the end of the day, before he went home, he sat down from a distance, and watch his masterpiece, then go home.

On one afternoon, another happy hour he was enjoying, unintentionally he listened some people's talking to each other, and he noticed the conversation almost becoming an argument.

In the beginning of the conversation, he was happy because everybody was unainmously complimenting the scluptuer. When the conversation moved to who was the sculptor, no one knew who did it. They guessed and spit out many names, but his name never came out.

He went home furious, because no one knew and said his name.

When he came back the next day, he brought his tool with him.

And, he carved his name across the chest of the grieving Mother.

This is the only sculpture with the sculptor's name on it.

If you go and stand close to it, you can see what he did. I'm talking anout his name.

I'm not a psychiatrist, but I'm sure he has personality disorder, obsessive comulsive type.

Why did he do such a stupid thing? He regreted later what he did, and pledged he will never do it again.

The answer is, because he has Personality disorder. Big time, personality disorder. They always regret what they did. Psychoes never regret.

Psyco.

In this world, there are many things that we can imitate, but cannot duplicate.

If we want to be someone in the past or present, we have to do our best as we can be. That is all we can do.

In our lisea, there are something that we can overcome, but at the same time, there are many things that we cannot.

We should know that we can pretend to be somebody but we cannot be that somebody. The only thing we can do is "pretend" or give up.

We can pretend to be Michael Jordan, but you cannot duplicate what Michael Jordan did. Do you think you can do it? O, please don't! Just be yourself.

We can pretend to be Wolfgang Amadeus Mozart, you cannot be Mozart.

We can pretend to be Michael Jackson, or Elvis Presley, but we can only immitate them.

You can pretend to be John F. Kennedy, but I know John Kennedy, you are not John Kennedy.

You want to be Leonardo Da Vinci, Van Goch or Michaelangelo, You can immitate them, that's all we can do.

But, in this case, if you think you can do better than Micaelangelo, of course, you are not he.

If you think you can do as good as, or better than Michaelangelo, that means you are suffering from Schizophrenia, paranoid type with grandiose delusion.

It happened in 1972, and the damage was caused by mentally disturbed Hungarian-born, Austrian young man, who thought he can do better than, or as good as Michaelangelo.

When he realized he is not him, and is far inferior than he, and he cannot be him, he came to St Peter's Basilica with the hammer.

He took a 15 blows to, and gave multiple damages to "Pieta". He was subdued by the other visitors.

Mary's left arm at elbow was broken, her nose, and few others were broken, too.

Many pieces was taken by the visitors near by at the time. Most of them are returned after heart-felt request by the Vatican, but her nose and few other pieces never returned.

After careful and meticulous restoration, "Pieta" is now sitting behind, and protected by a bulletproof glass panel, but you may not recognize it because the glass is so well-maintained, and so clean.

One of the characteristics of psycho is they never apologizes for what they have done, even after they committed a murder or multiple murder because they think they have done nothing wrong.

Costco

From mid February to the end of March, In Rome, it is pretty cold when the sun goes down.

You need a jacket which is very light, and very warm as well. Of course the price has to be reasonable, or not expensive, ie cheap.

A store which meets the above criteria is Costco.

There were so many stores like Costco that came and disappeared due to stiff competition, but this one seems to stay with us quite long time.

Costco's brand name is Kirkland, which means if certain items are very excellent in sales, they will produce their own items and sell it with a very reasonable price.

This is one of the big differences between Costco and other companies that came and gone.

So, I'm going to list several more reasons why Costco will remain my favorite store for years to come.

First.

It is the people, the employees.

The people who are working there look happy, or pleasant all the time.

When you get in, you are greeted with a smile. When you are leaving, you will see their smile. If you have any question, ypu will get the answer with a smile.

Most likely, they are being paid more than other stores. How much more? I do not know.

Second.

What is the most favorite fast food that Americans likes the most?

McDonald, Berger King, Wendy, Subway, Pizza, or What else? All wrong!

They put a bait in front of people's mouth that people cannot turn away.

The answer is Hot Dog. None of the above fast food restraunt sells hot dogs. I do not know the reason why, but maybe it is too easy to make it

Many people who are done with shopping, before they go home, they eat a hot dog, and then go home.

They make an excellent hot dog with 100% beef. Most of hot dogs are not made of 100% beef. On the top of the quality, the size is big. And then, for the bun, they use top quality of flours.

So, not only the taste is excellent, but also the price is more than reasonable.

Current price is 1$50 cents including all-you-can-drink pop. In the beginning it must have been just one dollar.

Hot dog is the best fast food, when you play golf.

And, when we go to the park for a picnic with families, with other fast foods, we always make sure to bring hot dogs.

We also put so called chili, which is ground beef, on the top of the hot dog, then, additionally boiled American cheese on the top of all those, then eat it.

Nothing can match this taste.

And then, they added pizza, which is my favorite, and few others to their menu.

Also this pizza is not a joke. Because they used the best quality of flours and other materials. The taste is excellent, and the price is excellent, too.

The taste is as good as any other pizza restraunt, and the price is uncomparable with other pizza.

With one big piece of pizza alone, it cost you only 1$50. and if you include all-you-can-drink pop it is 1$99. It will be just a little over 2$, that's all.

And, third.

When they build a Costco store, it looks like huge warehouse with plenty of parking space.

They build gas station at the corner of the parking area, and sell gasoline at the price cheaper than any other gas station.

So, the customers who came for shopping, put gas on their cars on the way out, if the tank is low or empty.

You can save 3 to 5 $ depending on the size of your gasoline tank.

Finally, just because I spoke so highly of Costco, I did not receive anything, or any bribery from CEO of Kirkland in Seatle, Washington.

The Church of Domine Quo Vadis

There is one more place we need to go.

If you go to Rome in a group with tour guide, you will not be able to see this place. Because this is not a place for tourist attraction. There is nothing artistically valuable, or historically important.

There is a small church in a walking distance from Catacombe, which is 40 or 50 minutes away from Terminale by bus or subway train.

The cemetary for the emperors or dignitaries are located inside of Rome, but the poor or the deserted are all buried in this Catacombe, which is one of the tourist attractions.

When you go to Catacombe, just remember this church is in a walking distance. If you have enough time, pay a visit for your own curiosity.

When you go into the labylinth of underground tunnel of Catacombe, you touch the wall, stony hard wall and thinking, "How this is possible? How this wall is standing? How this wall is still standing?"

I do not know the answer. I'm not an engineer or an architect. If you know the anaswer, share with me.

How big is this underworld ? Tour guide said no one knows how big.

This is perfect place for early Christians to have prayer meetings together without being caught by Roman soldiers.

Even the first Pope was buried here temporarily after he was crusified, somewhere in the tunnel of Catacombe, then moved to current buriel site, below the altar of St Peter's Basilica.

Ordinary guy Nero

Long, long time ago,

In Hollywood, there was an actor, who was very handsome, and tall, more handsome and taller than Clark Cable.

His name is Robert Taylor. One of the memorable movie that he made was "Quo Vadis."

When Peter recognized his crucified teacher in the early morning darkness, frightened Peter cried out, "Domine Quo vadis!"

The movie title came from what Peter said out of panic.

In that movie, like many other movies or TV stories, emotionally unstable Nero set the fire in the city of Rome, then blame it to the Christians to avoid the responsibility.

In many other movies, including this one, Nero was depicted as a leader, a middle-aged man, emotionally so unstable that he enjoyed watching the innocent people, the Christians, dying horribly either burn to death, or be killed by the starved beasts.

He, Nero, was, and still is a typical example of what will happen to a person who is intellectually unfit, and emotionally unstable, becomes the leader of the world, or the leader of the Roman Empire.

Maybe he was emotionally unstale, and Intellectually unfit in his later life, or after he became Emperor, but as far as I know, he was an average guy you can see among your friends or cousins.

Nero was only 16 years old, when he became the Emperor, and then when he killed himself being afraid of captured and executed by his own soldiers, he was only 29 years old, not even 30.

Actually, he was born to be perfectly normal, average, and ordinary person. Just like you or me, he liked to sing. He must have had a good, or excellent singing voice.

Sometimes, he composed his own song. Yes, he was a singer and song writer. He liked to sing his own song.

If he was born in modern time America, he would have been a singer and song writer like John Denver or Bob Dylan, who lived happy life, made others happy with his songs, and would havwe won a Nobel Prize.

But, the difference between him and us or Jonn Denver and Bob Dylan happened to be he happened to have super-intelligent, super-smart, super-energetic soccer mom as his mother.

As you can imagine, like we have seen it modern time in twenty first century, if a leader becomes a leader solely with the help of someone, the person, or many times the people who made him the leader become the leader behind the leader, if the leader is intellectually immature.

So, he became the leader of the Roman Empire. The Empire is not run by the Emperor, But, by the person who made him to be Emperor, to be exact, by the mother of the Emperor.

Anyway, as he grows older, he starts feeling threatened by this dominant, domineering mother. He becomes paranoid about his own mother, such an ambitious person that she herself might want to become an Emperor, or Emperess(?) maybe, someday, what if it is soon? When is it going to be? What if tomorrow?

Like any other average person, finally he make up his mind to eliminte the dominant figure, hovering over his head, telling him what to do and not to do all the time.

So, he takes an action on her, before she takes an action on him.

As you can imagine, if a person is a singer and song writer, he or she is a environmentalist. And, so is Nero.

City of Rome was flooded with people from everywhere. Even before Nero became Emperor, City of Rome was crowded not only with people but also with housing, next to each other, and on the top of each other. There were all kinds of symtoms and signs that Rome was becoming slumn, or already became slumn. When there is a fire, it is extremely difficult to put out the fire.

And, Nero, the environmentalist, who mentioned from time to time that City of Rome need to be rebuilt to prevent a disaster from happening.

"Domine, Quo vadis"

Indeed, there was a fire, a big fire that burnt the City of Rome for 3 days and nights.

In the movie, Nero was enjoying watching the the fire on the top of his palace.

But, in reality, he was in panic because the fire at that time was too big to handle. The only thing that the citizens of Rome was able to do was wathing the fire burning.

At the same time, a rumor was spreading out to the people much worse than the fire itself, which was the Emperor was the one who set the fire to clean up the dirty City of Rome.

Nero was so desperate to do something to defend himself that he was facing two petential disaters simultaneously. For the fire, he had nothing else to do but to watch it helplessly like anybody else. For the rumor, someone gave him an idea to put out the fire of rumor instanteously.

Blame it to the jews, the Christians. They came to Rome after their leader was executed by his own people.

At the time of Nero, the Christians were, or have been already the object of ever deepening hatered.

Because, they refuse to serve in the military, like every citizen of Roman Empire has to do, and is doing. Romans took a great pride in to be a soldier of their own country

Christians, also, refuse to pay the tax, like every citizen of Roman Empire has to do, and is doing. Christians send their tax(?) to the Temple in Jerusalem.

They refuse to recognize the Roman Empire as their own country. Instead, when they are together, they pray to their God to send their leader back to earth, who died not too long ago, and establish new kingdom.

So, Nero sends out his soldiers, starts executing Christians in public.

This is the time, when Peter, the next leader of the Christians decides to avoid the persecution of Roman Empire, by running away from Rome to save his life.

When his followers got caught on the street, and executed by being burnt, and being eaten by hungry beasts, he chose to save his own life.

So, on one night when everybody was fast asleep, he put every thing he owns and all of his family in a wagon, and leaves Rome.

When he was passing a hill nearby Catacombe, It must have been very early in the morning.

From Rome to that point, it took 40 to 50 minute in a subway train, he was on foot. We can safely say that it was very early morning the sun was about to come out.

He might have been thinking whether he should take a break.

At that moment, he saw a person coming from opposite direction. The person was tall like his teacher, but he told himself, "No, no way, he is the one." Shaking his head, "He could not be!"

As the distance between the two got closer, Peter recognized immediately who that young man was.

Apparently, it was not at night. It was not during the day.

If it was in the middle of the night, they would not have recognized each other. They would have passed by each other.

If it was bright day light, Peter would have recognized his teacher fron a distance, ran away from him, and hide where his teacher could not find. Peter is well known to us that he ran away from his teacher and hide to save his life more than once.

I think Jesus chose the time of morning darkness, not pitch black or broad day light.

Otherwise, the meeting between the two would not have occured. The most important meeting ever in the history of Christianity would not have happened.

That is why timing is everything in our lives. Momentum is so important.

When the two came so close to each other, almost face to face each other, they recognized each other.

As usual, out of panic, Peter crys out, "Domine, Quo Vadis."

He does not ask who he is first, why he is here, or where he came from. Out of all of those questions, he was concerned about the direction the most.

"Where are you going?"

Out of the free-will, and out of no where, Peter chose this question, the most important and the most famous question in the history of Christianity, without thinking.

We do not not know how long they talk to each other.

But, we do know the rest of the story.

There is a small church, not far from the road where they met on that early morning, although we do not know the exact spot.

The road where they met was built by the Emperor, Appius Claudius Caeus in 312BC, one of the road leading to Rome.

In Latin, the name is "Via Appia Antica", In Italian, Via Appia, in English, Appian Way.

This road is also famous, and of course Hollywood made a movie named "Spartacus."(BC 111-71)

When he revolted against Roman Empire, even though he was winning and victory after victory, he knew he cannot defeat Roman Emperial Army in the long run.

He makes a careful escape plan. He made a deal with the owner of many ships to escape to far away across the sea, a place where Roman soldiers cannot find them.

But, the deal broke off by the ship owner, who was afraid of stiff retaliation by the Romans.

He died in the battle near the Appian Way, and those who were captured, brought to this road. Thousands of the captured were executed by crusfixition on the crosses lined up on both sides of the road.

Spartacus died on BC71 at the age of 30, and his countless men were also died on the cross on BC71.

Almost 100 years later, at the age 30, Jesus also died on a cross, exactly the same way Spartacus' men died.

On that road, Appian Way, there is a small church, not fancy, definitely not tourist attraction.

But, if you choose to go inside, you will see a pair of footprints in a marble stone, which was said to be the footprints of jesus that appreared after the incident of the famous meeting.

It is a copy, the original is kept in somewhere else.

CHAPTER V.

WATER

Let me begin with the definition of the best water for our body.

Certainly, the quality has to be good, clean and uncontaminated chemically and boilogically, etc.

We are lucky enough to have good water around us. Especially, living in Michigan, right next to the Great Lakes.

But, in this world, there are many countries, many people who have no choice but to drink less than good water. It is very important to have good water. And, furthermore we have to make this good water the best water for us if possible. That is the main goal of this chapter.

I do not have any magical ability to turn less than good water into good, and then into the best water.

I do not have the magic power to turn the less than good water into the best water. All I can do is to make good water into the best.

This is my magic. From good to the best.

In this chapter, the main issue that I want to talk about is the best water.

This is how.

Like any other things in our lives, making the best from the good also depends on timing.

The timing has to be good.

The best water in this world is the water that I drink when all the cells of my body needed the most. The plain water next to me is the best water, when my cells, are thirsty, ie dehydrated, not my tongue or my lips.

Why not when I feel thirsty? I drink when I feel thirsty.

Wrong! Dead wrong! Because it is too late.

This is why. By the time you feel thirsty in your mouth or in your brain, your cells are already dehydrated, which means you are opening, and entering the doorstep of dying or death of your cells, plain and simple.

By the time you feel thirsty, by the time your lips, your tongue feel dry, it is already too late.

Of course, the quality of the water is important.

But, in oder to make good water the best, it is timing. Like anything else in our lives, timing is the key.

You have to drink water before you feel thirsty. This is the key.

Most of us are looking for a good water, and most of us do have good water. From now on, we have to learn, and train ourselves to make the good to the best.

However, we cannot look inside of our body, especially we cannot put a microscpe into the cell, there is no other way to tell when our cells need water.

So, unlike any other chapter, in this chapter, let me tell you the conclusion first, which is;

"Drink wisely" which means, "Drink a little, and drink frequently" before we feel thirsty.

We are in trouble if we drink too little, or drinking water too much, we are in trouble, too.

The only, and the best way to drink water is "a little, and frequent."

The water content of our body is a bit over 2/3, up to 70%, and only 1/3, or 30% is not water. That means if a person is weighing 150 lbs, only 50 lbs is not water, meaning 100 lbs is water. Just imagine how much water we are dealing with if a person is weighing over 300 lbs.

So, to be exact, when we fade away, majority of our body has to go bak to the water. Only small portion of our body goes back to the dust. It is more accurate when we say, "water to water" rather than "dust to dust." We go back to the water more than to the "dust.

Water is so important to our body, that in near future we will all fight for the drinking water rather than oil. Actually it is already happening inside of US, not far from us.

I live in Michigan, near Great Lakes, where we do not hear much about water shortage, or drought and so on.

But, many States like California, Nevada, Arizona, Texas, etc are going through serious water shortage every year, sometimes they request asistance, but the governers of Great Lakes decline each time. Even Federal Government, or the President of USA can not order these States what to do.

Silent war is already going on inside US, not to mention outside of America.

In my experience, the waters from the Great Lakes is the best water amomg all the good waters.

And, deep in the Canadian Rocky Mountains, we can have a rare opportunity to meet glacier ice water.

Over thousands years, tens of thousand years, hundreds thousand years, or millions years ago, heavy snow after heavy snow, accumulation after accumulation, develop into glacier, and then over the glacier, another one, and another one, and another one.

Due to the weight and the gravity, giant glacier is pushed down little by little. When it is pushed down to a certain level to hit the temperature of melting point, the glacier starts melting.

And, it forms a small creek. If you put your hand in this creek, you will lose your feeling of your hand within a few seconds.

When I drink this water, once it goes in, I have the feeling that not only it is cleaning up my contaminated guts, but also it is cleaning up my dirty mind.

I hope all of the readers of this book have this experience, drinking the best of the good. You will have once in a lifetime experience that you will never forget.

What is good water?

We can safely say well cleaned, uncontaminated water would be good enough. It would be better if the water is boiled and cooled. Not too cold, not too hot. I recommend to drinks like green tea which is proven to contain high content of antioxident.

Then, what is bad water?

The worst example is those water with alcohol, also called whiskey, beer, and so on. If you drink this kind of water wisely, it can be good for our body. But, if you drink this water unwisely, it will be bad for body and mind for sure. We all know that. Also bad is the water with caffeine, such as coffee, and caffenated soda, etc. Recently, it concerns me that we see in commercial more and more the water called 'Energy Drink."

In the recent studies, researchers report that too hot water may be harmful to our body, although more studies needs to be done.

In my opinion, too cold water may not be good to our body either, more specifically to our stomach.

I do not recommend people drinking soda, such as cola with ice as often seen in the advertizement. If you want, or have to drink cola with ice, drink it extremely slow.

Likewise, in the hot summer sun, I do not encourage people drinking ice cold beer with a big smile in the beer commercial.

You may feel good today, but certainly your stomach will complain to the owner later on.

What is thirst? Why do we feel thirsty?

When we feel thirsty, it comes with subtle physical change at the same time. It is not just a feeling. Our mouth as well as tongue and lips gets dry. Of course skin gets dry too.

When we have certain conditions, we will end up having serious illness, or disease related with water. Usually water-related conditions comes and goes very quick. If you do not treat the patient immediately or in time, you can lose your patient real easy.

We can think of two conditions.

One is we have too much water in our body, and the other is opposite, too little water. When we are talking about water in our body, we have to keep in mind electrolytes at the same time. So, in the textbook, we call this condition Fluid and Electrolyte Imbalance.

In a condition called 'fluid overload', either we drink too much, or we do not eliminate fluid in time.

Most of the time, with kidney disease, or heart disease, we end up with serious problem like Chronis Renal Failure.

And now, the other extreme, fluid depleted or dehydrated.

When we have a condition that we eliminate fluid, or water too much. And then we go into a condition called "Dehydration," which is one of "Fluid and Electrolyte Imbalance."

In case of dehydration, based on severity, we classify this condition into 3, which is mild, moderate, and severe. In a case of severe dehydration, people can die, particularly in pediatric populations even with simple diarrhea itself newborn babies die easily. This condition is one of pediatric emergencies, and Pediatrician's nightmare.

Here, what we are going to discuss about is mild case of dehydration as a result of not drinking enough water, with which we are not dealing with life or death situation, but it can be serious and potentially dangerious with geriatric populations.

Unfortunately, our body does not have early warning system of any dehydration. Instead, we have late warning system, which means, by the time we get the warning signal, ie thirst, or feeling thirty, it is already too late.

By the time, our cells cry outloud that they are thirsty and dehydrated, and the desperate message goes to our brain, then our tongue, and lips, our cells are already on the verge of death, or some of our cells are no longer alive because of dehydration. And yet, most of us ignore even this late warning signal of thirst or being thirsty.

So, to prevent this preventable, unnecessary tragedy from happening is to drink small amount of water as frequently as possible.

I grew up in a culture where the seniors, mostly parents, encourage not to drink water. They discourage water drinking. Most likely reason for this culture might be originated from bed wetting at night. Always my parents made sure to tell me, "Don't drink before you go to bed!!!!"

When we are having a serious meeting either business or religious, it does not look good, if somebody disrupt the flow of the meeting to go to the bathroom.

Earlier, I emphasized that our body has twice as much water than the solid portion. So, I cannot hardly emphasize more about the enormous importance of water in our body. Everything goes in our body mixed with water or water alone, and comes out mixed with water such as sweat, urine and stool.

In a way, our body is like a water baloon with some "dust(?)" inside.

So, again, I have to say we have to drink a little, and as frequent as possible. I do not know how little is little, and how frequent is frequent. These are all subjective. Your little can be too much for me. Somebody's too much can be too little for me. Your frequent can be not frequent for me. Somebody's frequent can be not frequent for me.

This has to be individualized. You have to come up with your own amount of water, and frequency. I have to come up with my little amount of water and frequency.

Because we cannot see inside of our cells to tell how much and when the cells are dehydrated.

It is not good, and I do not recommend drinking large amount of water at a time. Whatever the reason is, when we are thirsty, ie dehydrated, we drink a lot. In this situation, I would still recommend drink a little and more frequently.

Why? If we drink a large amount of water at a time, exactly like a baloon, our stomach has to expand, the wall of our stomach has to stretch. This is when our stomach pumps out the digestive enzymes and gastic acid. In this situation, our stomach has no defense from the acid, we have nothing to neutralize the acid that our own stomach produced. The gastric acid will hurt your stomach wall real bad.

When and if you eat, the food you ate will act as antacid. The food itself will act as antacid that neutralizes the acid.

So, It is more dangerous to have gastric acid pouring out after drinking a lot of water at a time than after eating a big meal because the food is neutralizing the acid to some extent.

In general, this is the reason why beer drinkers are having more stomach problem and/or pancreatic problem than whiskey drinkers, who generally are having more liver problem.

I do agree that little bit of alcohol is good for our body and mind, but I rarely see many of us have the ability to control the amount of alcohol once we start drinking.

When we drink alcohol, we often see 3 group of people. First group: People drink alcohol. People control alcohol. And, next Second group: Alcohol drinks alcohol. Alcohol controls people. Then, Third group: Alcohol drinks people. Both human and alcohol go out of control, and no one knows who is in charge. Alcohol says, "I'm in charge," and control human.

I do not understand why people are competing how much they can drink.

Even though I was born with no to a little alcoholic gene that I rarely drink alcohol more than I want, I have no problem people drinking alcohol to get high as much as they want.

But, I have a "big" problem with those people who drink more than as much as they want and being called "alcoholic" being controlled by alcohol.

Why do you have to be called alcoholic ?

As I said, I have no problem with people, drinking alcohol as much as to get "high", ie to feel "good." or feel "better."

I do have big problem with people who have to drink more than as much as they need, either to show off their manhood such as in college campuses, or to express their anger or for no reason whatsoever, etc

If someone need the help of ancohol, other reasons than to get "high", ie to feel "good," he or she needs the help of psychiatrists, psycho;ogists, priests, or ministers, not alcohol.

It's about time to conclude.

We are made of, or made from water. And, when we are being made, we were in the water.

Then, after awhile when the time comes, we all go back to water. Only 1/3 of me go back to the "dust."

So, when or if we lose certain amount of, or just a little bit of water, we can get sick easily, and/or we can die easily.

Just look at a newborn baby, she or he can die real easy with a simple diarrhea only, which is the worst nightmare of pediatricians, and/or pediatric residents.

For the grown ups, we think we have a early warning signal aka thirst, or feeling thirsty, which is very unreliable that by the time we feel thirsty, it is already too late at celluar level.

In the ordinary situation, when we have drinking water around us, we rarely die because of dehydration only. But, in the worst scenario, we can die due to dehydration when the water intake stops and/or too much water loss.

In this chapter, we are discussing about water, in ordinary setting. We are not going to die just because we are thirsty.

We are trying to make a Good Water turn into the Best Water for me or for allof us.

Whici is; Drink wisely.

"DRINK A LITTLE, AND FREQUENTLY AS POSSIBLE !!!"

Chapter VI.

Tutangkamen, aka "King Tut"

When you visit Cairo, the capital city of Egypt, you will go to the Museum of Egyptian Antiquities, aka Museum of Cairo, one of the must-see tourist attractions in Egypt.

At the entrance of the Museum, you have to give up all of your photographic equipment, and then receive a ticket to retrieve your belongs when you leave.

There are many places where you are not allowed to take photos, but this one is the only rare place that you have to turn in your photo equipment.

Once you get in, it is not allowed for anyone to talk loud inside, especially for the tour guides to speak loud to his, or her group. So, our tour guide told us to sit down on the stair of the the first floor, and explains about what to see, what we should not miss, and so on.

Feeling a bit upset, because you cannot take any pictures, and you cannt not talk to each other, either, if your voice goes high.

My freedom of speech, and my freedom of recording are well restricted. I do not understand why so many places are restricting photos.

What kind of damage does it give to paintings, sculptures, antiques, and so on by taking pictures without flashes? Or even with flashes. Some scientists have to do a research about what is potential damage about being the object of photos. If taking pictures can cause damage to the life-less object, what about us? We are living humans.

Anyway, while listening to the guide, most of us, especially very sensitive minded ladies of our group cannot help but having a few tears in their eyes.

After the tour guide, who made us sure to look at the flowers on the sarcophagus of King Tut that was given by his wife, the Queen, finished his speech, we were all free to go around wherever we want to go.

In the 4 story building, it is quite big building, if 2 or 3 of the 4 floors are filled with, and came from one person's burial site, from one tomb, who is going to believe that?

This is excellent example of how powerful, and how rich Pharaoh can be. Pharaoh had absolute political power, military leader, and absolute religious authority, who were at same level with god, and he owned everything in the country.

That is why the name, Pharaoh Tutankhamun, meaning "Living image of Amun" Amun is Sun god.

So, the Pharaoh had three absolute powers in one individual.

First,

Like any other leader, he is on the top of everyone on the country. He is the country. Sometimes he designantes this power to someone else, such as his son, or loyal follower. Even so, he still holds the ultimate power.

Second,

Simutaneously, he is military leader. He is the commander in chief. The difference is, when there is a war, he does not stay behind. He, himself, goes to the war, not his son or his general. Even at war, he always stays in the front, not behind. Even if Pharaoh dies in the battlefield, they never say, "Our Pharaoh died while fighting the enemy", because Pharaoh does not die. God never dies. You cannot find in any records documenting Pharaoh died as a result of a disease, a war, or old age, etc, because he is God, not human being.

Another difference compared to other country is Egypt, ie Pharaoh, had standing military force, ready to go to war all the time. Not like the rest of the countries, having generals and few elite force in a peaceful period, then, when there is a war, ordinary people become the main force voluntarily or involuntarily.

Egypt was opposite. They had an army ready to go to war any time. Generals and soldiers, the war professionals, always ready to kill enemies. Financially, they can afford to have, keep and maintain a huge standing army physically and mentally ready.

Third,

As mentioned above, he is God. He is not human. No further explanation is necessary what kind of power he has. He is the one and only highest priest as well, who does not die.

Fourth,

Egyptians were rich, which means Pharaoh was rich, who owned the country. The River Nile gave the Egyptians more than enough wealth to become the strongest country in that part of the world.

Two rivers from south, one is from Ethiopia, another one is from Kilimanzaro, becomes long and long Nile river, which overflow twice a year that brings to Egypt with rich soil. They have plenty of harvests of grains twice a year. That's why Egypt could afford to have a standing army, always ready to fight, who were making their living by fighting.

So, when famine spread to Middle East, and even in Southern Europe, people come to Egypt to get the food, or move and stay in Egypt untill the crisis is over. To the people of Middle East, or Eastern Europe, Egypt was filled with peace, and abundent foods.

Even for the political reasons, Jesus came down to Cairo with his parents, and lived few to many years in Egypt. We do not know exactly how long the holy family stayed in Egypt.

Not to mention that there is a threat from other countries, even in peaceful periods, Pharaoh takes his army and goes to war twice a year, once to the the north such counties in middle east, the most frequent target was Lebanon, and once to the south, such as Ethiopia, and Sudan, and so on.

We can not compare the civilization of Egyptian culture with any other cultures in the history of humanity, because Egyptian had their own letter, language, unique art, military system that other cultures did not have.

The civilization of Mesopotamian cuture is almost a thousand years longer than Egyptian culture, but Egypt had to be far superior to any other cultures in terms of national wealth, military strength, religious authority, etc.

Geographically, Egypt is well proteced from outside enemies.

Occasionally, being invaded from the north, and the south, that is the reason why Pharaoh brings his army to the north once, and to the south once annually to show off the strength of Egyptian military.

To the east, there is Red Sea, then Saudi Arabia. Saudi Arabia is a country of desert, and does not have big trees to make good ships. So, Saudis do not have strong Navy.

To the west,

There is Sahara Desert, protecting Egypt. The desert is protecting Egypt.

From the north,

Occasionally, Egypt was invaded from north. They put the Egyptian military on the northern border, and further more once a year, Pharaoh brings his army to north, and make sure they cannot even think about invading Egypt. So, throughout the hitory of Egypt, up untill the era of Cleopartra, Egypt did not have any serious threat from the north. Maybe, once or twice.

From the south,

Of course, Pharaoh brings his army annually to the South, such as Sudan or Ethiopia.

But, the problem, the headache is defending, protecting the border. Of course, the best defense is offense. That's what they do every year. But, it is practically impossible to go to war all the time. And, the southern border of Egypt is too wide and too long.

So, in addition to the annual offense, Ramses the Great constructs Abu Simbel on the top of rocky mountain at the southern border.

He builds huge, and giant statues of himself, and the Sun God, outside, and also inside of the cave.

And the next to his temple, he builds another temple dedicated to his wife, the Queen.

So, he constructs two gigantic temples, with huge statues at the very strategic spot, where the enemies coming from south have to pass the Abu Simbel.

If you stand in front of this structure, immediately you will feel, that they are big and huge, and you are small and tiny.

As a result, if you are the enemy of Egypt, and you are the leader of the invading force, immediately you are going to lose the fighting will, which will disappear at once. And, you will get homesick right away. You will think about not being able to see your famoly left behind. You want to go home dropping your weapon to the ground, and turn around.

But, as a tourist, as a visitor, no sooner you stand in front of the gigantic structure, than you cannot help but feeling your heart, your mind becomes empty, and get humbled by the great achievement of my fellow human being, although we were born in a different time and different place.

Even though I visited many different places, and saw many structures of small and huge, when I stood in front, my jaw dropped to the ground, and I could not find it even though I wanted to shut my mouth.

Twice a year, on a particular day in the spring, and in the fall, when the sun rises, the ray of sunshine comes into the cave, and drops at right shoulder of Ramses the Great.

According to the tour guide, on those two days, myriad of tourists come to Abu Simbel the day or 2 days before, many of them are camping on the ground in front of the entrance, and wait for the time.

In fact, the arts of stone carving originated from Egypt, to the Greek who leaned from Egyptians, then the Greek spread to the Romans and to the rest of the Europe, and the world. Especially, Alexander the Great was the one who spread this art form from Europe to India. Then, from India to China, And From China to Korea. Finally, from Korea to Japan.

I still remember that we used to buy a seal like a postage stamp from school when I was in the elementary school. It was an effort to save Abu Simbel from drowning ie going under water when Egyptian government of Nasser was building Aswan dam in the area of Abu Simbel. UNESCO was the one that organized the movement to save Abu Simbel.

They meticulously cut the mountain rock 1 meter by 1 meter by 1 meter, and moved to above the water level where they are now.

As a matter of fact, modern time Egyptians are not Egyptians. They are Arabics. Actually, the real Egyptians are from down south of Africa, followed up the water route of Nile river. Strictly speaking, they are Africans.

So, present time of Egypt, most of the so-called Egyptians are Moslem, who came down from Middle East, or further north country like Iran.

In the modern history, when someone becomes the president of Egypt, even though you do not know for sure whether you are an true Egyptian or not, he feels like or acts like a Pharaoh. What an irony we are looking at.

But, in the history of Egypt, many of the heroes in Europe, or Mediteranian region desperately wanted to become the Pharaoh of Egypt.

First of all, we can pick Alexander the Great of Macedonia.

His father, the King of Macedon, was assassinated, he was 20 year old, and took over the throne. He continued his father's battle, and defeated the mighty Persians, whose leader was the great king Darius III. (BC333)

Then, he goes to Egypt as a liberator, not as a conqueror, and become an Egyptian, to be Pharaoh of Egypt. As a field general, he never lost a single battle untill he dies at the age of 30. He was coming back from India. Egypt was, then, given to one of his trusted general, Ptolemy

So, for the next 300 years or so, untill the fall of Egyptian Empire, Egypt was ruled by the Greeks, not by Egyptians.

And, next

My favorite person in the history of Roman Empire, Julius Caesar, who became Pharaoh by marrying another Pharaoh, also the inventor of Nile River Cruise with Cleopatra, which we are doing it 2000 years later.

He was born in July of 100BC, assassinated by his fellow men on March of 44BC, who were afraid that Ceasar was becoming too powerful as one person.

He transformed single-handedly the Roman Republic to the Roman Empire, where one individual holds all the power as Emperor, instead of Senate, where many individuals shared the power.

As a military leader, he conquered and expand the territory to the modern day France and Belgium, and made Rome ever bigger than before, even stronger than before, and more importantly even safer than before.

As a political leader, with help of ever rising popularity of all of the Romans, he started eliminating his political opponents, and concentrating the power on one person, himself.

When Pompeyus, the leader of Republicans, head of main opposition of Caesar, fled to Egypt, Ceasar followed him. But, Pompeyus was alreadyassassinated by Cleopatra's brother, for fear that he might be blamed if Pompey was still alive.

By then, the entire world knew who has the ultimate power.

Two MIP(most important person, most influential person) in the history of humanity, of course, one is Jesus Christ, the other is Julius Caesar, who impacted immensely on people's lives then and even now, might have met each other in Egypt if Jesus was born a bit sooner.

Now, the super power of the world moved to the Roman Empire, not Egypt. The super power of Roman Empire was concentrated on one person, Julius Caesar.

By the time Caesar came to Egypt, he aleady became the most powerful man of the world. In Egypt, there was power struggle between the siblings, but the one who got the attention, and support of Caesar became the winner of power struggle.

Cleopatra, young, talented, intellegent, and beautiful becomes Pharaoh of Egypt.

In Rome, all the citizen of Rome were anxiously waiting for the triumphant return of their hero.

But, there was no sign of their hero to return, instead, all they were hearing was their hero got married to Egyptian Queen, and they were on honeymoon on the Nile River, the first Nile River Cruise or any cruise of the world history. It is political marrage for Cleopatra, who needed a powerful figiure behind her to govern her country. She was in her early 20s, and Caesar was in his 50s. We all know who is controlling who. We all know who is in charge. Romans knew better, and more than anybody else, and they are getting angry. But, instead of hating or angry at Caesar, Romans choose to hate Cleopatra. They began to destroy any statues or paintings if there is any. That was the reason why we do not see any of her face, or entire body painting or statues.

By the time their hero returned to Rome with Cleopatra, he beccame or was already, not only the Emperor of Roman Empire, but also Pharaoh of Egypt.

So, to the eyes of the patriotic Romans, Julius Caesar was not one of their own anymore. He has too much power, and wants to be God, and is already God. To ordinary Roman, he is too dangerous.

And, they do something that they regret right away, Ordinary people kill their God. Immediately they knew they did something really bad.

And,"You know the rest of the story."

And, third, who tried to be Pharaoh, but failed.

This individual is a French hero, whose name is Napoleon Bonaparte, born in 1769, and died in 1821.

After triumphant return from Italy, he planed to invade the England, which was his long time dream.

As his plan gets more practical, he realizes it is practically next to impossible thing to achieve, because he does not have decent naval forces to cross over the Channel, or the Strait of Dover, and invade the England, or to engage in naval warfare if necessary. He does not know much about a war at sea. And, the other reason is he is an artillary officer.

So, instead, he decided to invade Egypt to block the Suez canal, so that marchant ships or military vessels of England have to sail around the African continent to go India, and come back same route. His strategy was to give signficant blow to the economy of England, and wait untill the appropriate time to attack.

But, this was not the only reason that he wanted to occupy Egypt. He wanted to do exactly what his personal heroes, Alexander the Great, and Julius Caesar, did.

To be the Paraoh of Egypt.

At that time, he was only 29 years old. He was very ambitious man as we all know, and nothing's gonna stop him. He came to Egypt not only with his military force, but also with a bunch of non-militaty personels for the exact purpose unknown. He brought approximately 150 of scientists with him, of course, many archeologists and some are artists.

He goes to Egypt, forces out Turkish Military who was defending Egypt, and occupies Egypt briefly. It was only brief, because Admiral Nelson came to the rescue of Egypt from French occupation, because he knew the importance of Suez canal, militarily and economically.

But, as soon as Napoleon's Army occupied Egypt, they began huge exacavation, and collecting as many antiques as possible.

Soon, there was Admiral Nelson, Naval warfare genius, who recognized the seriousness of the blockade of Suez canal.

He, Admiral Nelson himself showed up with his fleet, and as a result, Napoleon's entire fleet sank to the bottom of the sea, which was later called "Battle of the Nile."

Napoleon had to escape to Paris, without achieving his biggest dream of his life, ie, becoming Pharaoh of Egypt.

Although his mission ended up with total failure, with help of extremely poor communication, and total lack of mass media, he received hero's welcome in Paris, because he told the country that he liberated Egypt with great military success. Then, to distract the people's attention away from failure in Egypt, he invade Russia, which happened to be the beginning his demise, his downfall.

By the way, about the time he was receiving hero's welcome, and marching through the streets of Paris, the rest of the troops and the scientists who were captured and became prisoners' of war by Nelson, were receiving as much humiliation as Napolen's hero's welcome.

They were ordered to give up and turn in to Nelson every antiques that they have collected, and excavated.

At the negotiation table, the commanding general representing French Army had no choice but to turn in everythig they had. Although he made an offer or request or plead to Nelson to keep the Rosetta stone that they found, Nelson was firm. Nelson was so firm that they were very lucky that they return to Paris without losing their lives.

Every item they collected including Rosetta stone, was given to Nelson, and brought to London, rather than Paris.

And, "you know the rest of the story." We all know that who the owner of the Rosetta stone is, and in what museum it is kept since then,

The history of Egypt, we know, began on 3100BC when Pharaoh Narmer united North and South Egypt.

So, Narmer built Old Kingdom, which lasted about 1000 years, then came the first Intermediate Period(BC2181-BC2049), and then came the Middle Kingdom(BC2134-BC1782), then came the Second Intermediate Period (BC1782-BC1650), and the last, comes the New Kigdom.

At the end of the New Kingdom, on BC332, Egypt was concquered by Alexander the Great, and was ruled by the Greek untill BC30, when Cleopatra, the last Pharaoh of Egypt, marries to Julius Caesar, who became the first Emperor of Roman Empire, and the last Pharaoh of Egypt.

Officialy, the history of Egypt ended BC32, but practically it ended in BC332.

At the peak of the New Kingdom, there was a Pharaoh whose name was Amenhotep IV, later he changed his name to Akhenaten (ruled Egypt BC1350-1334), which means "Effective for Aten." He is the father of "King Tut" who is the main character of this chapter.

Unlike the tradition, he married to a commoner, Nefertiti, who was the most beautiful woman in the history of Egypt. Besed on the record, some aecheologists claims she is more beautiful than Cleopatra.

When he changed his name, he began to preach there is only one god, "Aten." Typically, Egypt has been a country of multiple god, very progressive and open minded society.

All of a sudden, people of Egypt were told by their living god, that there is only one god, Aten.

But, there was no bloody conflict, between one god, Aten, and the rest of gods. They maintained peaceful co-existence, which happens to be entirely different from what is happening in present world of 21 century.

Those who believe and claim that there is only One god and nothing else, must go back to the history of Egypt, and learn from Akhnaten, the most generous, and open-minded, one and only religious leader of entire human history, from the beginning till the present day of humanity.

There was no political, social, or religious turmol between the two, Polytheism vs monotheism.

He had all the power and authority to surpess and wipe out other religions, but chose not to. He accepted the existance of other gods.

It appears that God, and the Pharaoh as well, allowed his people to worship other gods, other than Aten, the one and only, his god. God, the Pharaoh, allowed his people the freedom to worship other god.

This is absolutely unacceptable, not allowed in any religions in the 21 century.

Then, he build a new holy city, and the capital, 200 miles away from Thebes, in the middle of Sahara desert, Tell el Amarna. He moves the capital city with his followers, from Thebes to the new city that he build with his followers, those who believe in Aten like he does.

This is a revolution. One and only true revolution. No one put into jail, and no one died, not even one single soul, without a single drop of blood.

Indeed, aecheologists call this entire event Amarna Revolution.

There are many revolutions in the history of the world, but, there is no revolution as radical as this one, and yet no one died.

Again, this single event shows exactly how powerful a Pharaoh is.

He had 3 daughter with Nefertiti, the most beautiful woman in the history of Egypt.

He had a son, Tutankhamen, in his later life with his minor wife, Kiya,

Unfortunately, Akhenaten died when King Tut was only 8 years old.

Tutankhamen becomes Pharaoh of Egypt at the young age of 8, and then marries with his 2 years older half sister, Ankhesenamen. According to the tradition of Egyp, in order to be a ligitimate Pharaoh, you have to marry the first daughter of Pharaoh. This is the most ligitimate way to become a Pharaoh.

Although the marriage within the royal family does have a advantage, but simultaneously has invisible disadvantages. If you marry within the royal family, the power remains within the family. But, if you marry within the family, it has high probability to have genetic mutation or genetic defects, as a result, high incidence of stillbirth, genetic disease and hereditary disease.

By the way, what does he know about religion or politics as a 8 year old boy ?, and what does she know about religion or politics as a 10 year old girl?

Egypt had Pharaoh, the King and the Queen, but the country was ruled by the king's adviser, the prime minister, Aye, who moved the capital back to Thebes.

The young couple grow up together like a sibling, though practocally they are half brother, and half sister with same father.

Apparently, they had two babies, but they appeared to be stillborn.

Then, Tutankhamen dies suddenly.

For the cause of his death, there are 2 theories; One is due to infection, gangrene of his leg. And, the other is murder. Killed by someone.

First, He died of some kind of infectious disease unteatable with ancient medicine that they had to watch him to die slowly. Most likely cause of his death was a massive gangrene of lower extremity due to wound infection inflicted in a fight with enemies, or during strenuous physical activities.

The scientists who investigated to find the cause of his death, now agreed that there was no evidence of skull fracture, or hematoma inside his skull based on X-Rays and CAT scans.

Second, King Tut was too young to govern Egypt, the superpower of nothern Africa, Middle East.

Quite naturally, the Pharaoh's adviser, the prime Minister, Aye, is the one who controls everything. He is the ruler of Egypt behind the young Pharaoh.

As King Tut grew older, it is just a matter of time that he has to give up all the power he had back to the fast growing, young Pharaoh.

So, the Pharaoh's fate is at the hands of his "best" man. He plans to kill the Pharaoh, then forces the Queen to marry him. Then, he announces to the nation that he, himself, is the legitimate Pharaoh, then no one will object the God. Of course, the country will never believe, the Pharaoh was dead, or killed by someone. They will believe the young Pharaoh went to the next world. In the history of any country, when the King is betrayed by his "best" man, the King is most vulnerable.

So, as he planned, he commits the perfect crime, and bury the young Pharaoh in a hurry. Usually, Pharaoh's funeral lasts at least few years. But, his funeral must have lasted few months only.

During the funeral, the Queen goes to Nile river, pick up beautiful flowers with her own hands. She lays the flowers on the top of King Tut's sarcophagus.

When King Tut's tomb was found untouched in 1922 by Howard Cater, people found the mummified flowers on the top of King Tut's sarcophagus.

When the King Tut's body was becoming mummified, the flowers also became mummified with him. Most likely, the queen's grieving heart of the young Queen became mummified with her husband.

When tourists see this mummified flowers, people beome a bit emotional, including myself.

Now, the young Queen has to marry the old Prime Miinister, but was very afraid of him. Because she knows who murdered her husband, and why. Just imagine how scary it would be for the young woman, about 20 years old, who killed her young husband, and the person, more than 60 years old, wants to marry her ?

How do the archelolgists find out about this plot? There is a evidence, not direct, but indirect.

She sends a letter to the King of the Hittites, saying she is willing to marry to one of his sons, the Prince, which the King agrees. He accepts the offer that his son will be the next Pharaoh of Egypt.

But, the Prince never shows up in Egypt. The Prince and his soldiers also murdered by a group of strong army in civilian clothes in the middle of the night, when they were crossing the border.

Because this event was written in the history of the country Hittites.

Unfortunately, he died young.

But, he got lucky after he died. Because, no one tooched his burial site.

There is not a single Pharaoh's tomb, except King Tut's. There are so many Pharaohs in the history of Egypt, and so many Pharaoh' tombs. But, no Pharaoh's tombs are untouched except this one.

The very explanation for the reason that we, oe archeologists can think of, as some of archeologists speculate, is when a Pharaoh's tomb was built and completed, before long the very people who built the tomb who know what's in the tomb, come back and take away the valuables.

And then, when the people's interest, or curiosity enhanced by the discovery of the Rosetta Stone, exacavation and collection of Egyptian antiques became much more rampant than ever.

Ever since the fall of Cleopatra, Egypt was owned by Roman Empire, more specifically by Emperor of Rome, then by the Muslims from Arab countries, which means Egypt was a country, but without a government of their own.

So, any countries or any persons who come to Egypt and collect the antiques, automatically, quite naturally become the owner of whatever they collected.

CHAPTER VII

ZANTAC

Wake up in the morning, take one Baby Aspirin, and before you go to bed, take one Zantac.

Start your day with Aspirin, and finish your day with Zantac.

I'm going to explain the reason why we should take Aspirin in the chapter of "Aspirin" But, in this chapter, I'll explain why we should take one Zantac.

The reason why I advocate about Zantac is to protect our poor stomach, the most abused organ in our body. Unlike other organs, being abused the most, but never complains. Since we cannot witness the moment of abuse, and barely feel the consequencies of abuse, untill we face the real tragedy of the abuse by the owner, the abuse will continue.

We, humans, are the only animal, who eats 3 times a day, sometimes more than 3 times a day.

Also, we, humans, are the only animal, who eats not only for survival of our species, but also for ths pleasure of food's taste itself. It is same in the issue of sex, not only for the survival, but also for the pleasure itself.

And yet, we, humans, are the only animal, who cooks before we eat the food to make it taste better.

So, depending on the culture, we put so many different ingredients to the food.

Since I was born, and raised in Korea, I have no other choice to talk about Korean foods.

I'm going to be honest about when I talk about Korean food.

Generally speaking Korean foods are one of the best healthy food of all, if not the best.

So, seeing is believing. Just go to Korean restoraunt, and take a look.

Generally, the main dishes are high quality of cooked rice along with well boiled soup, sometimes many hours boiled soup from bone and meat.

And then you will see many and all different side dishes, from which you will absorb all different nutrition. I'm talking about all the vitamins and minerals. Count the number of side dishes, and compare with any other oriental reatraunts, or any reatraunt.

Tell me if there is any ethnic food, that serves more side dishes than Korean reatraurant.

Simply, among oriental restraunts, Chinese or Japanese included, how many side dishes do you see?

And, if you like any of the side dishes, if and when you finish one side dish, ask to give you more, the servers are more than happy to give you more. There is no extra charge for additional side dishes. Do not hesitate to ask more side dishes if you like. Sometimes, even before you ask more, if the waitress recognizes your side dish is empty, she will ask you if you want to have that particular side dish more.

That is the core of Korean culture that it will be given to you, before you ask what you want. You do not need to say anything, just make an eye contact with the waitress. That's all.

So far, I mentioned good side of Korean food. It is impossible to list all the good aspects of Korean food and culture.

Next, bad aspects of Korean food, and food culture. This is how Koreans are assaulting their own stomach. There are 3 ways of assaulting our stomach.

First, the way the food is prepared.
Second, the quantiy of one meal.
Third, the speed

First, the way the food is prepared.

The food is spicy and salty. This is main character of Korean food. The saltier and the spicyer, the better the taste will be.

I do not mean to say all the Korean food are spicy and salty, and only the Korean foods are salty and spicy. There are many other country's food, which are more salty, and more spicy than Korean food. At the same time, certainly there are many Korean foods that are not salty and spicy.

In terms of spicy food, a friend of mine from India gave me a treat with very high quality of curry.

Yes, indeed. It was so spicy that it burned and then numbed my tongue and lips for hours. It was one of the most, or may be ths most spicy food I ever had in my life. I can definitely, and respectably say that the spicyness of Korea food is no match for the spicyness of Indian food.

In terms of spicyness of food, I'd like to talk about halopino of Turkey, the spicyest and hottest halopino of all. In my experience, Korean halopino is no match against Mexican halopino, and Mexican halopino is no match against Turkeyish halopino.

Because, I have never seen a person passing out, literally losing consciousness while eating halopino except this one, Turkeyish halopino

It happened few years ago, when I was traveling Turkey in a group tour.

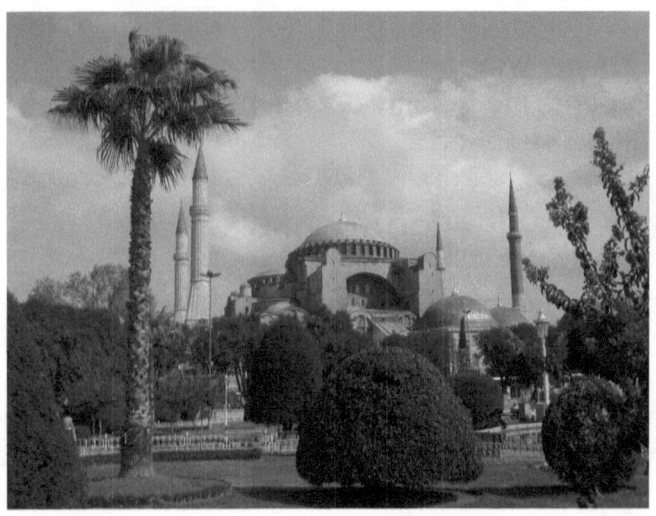

One day, at the end of the day, we arriived our hotel for the dinner and much needed rest and sleep. It was one of the best hotel in the city. There was live music to stimulate our appetites. The dinner was a buffet. It was wonderful.

There was so much to enjoy. Big piece of beef stakes, fresh and crispy vegetable, and so on.

I picked up a few of very good and innocent looking halopino.

Unfortunately, also fortunately, I started my dinner with halopino, and the moment I crushed the halopino, and even before chewing, I felt a burning sensation in my mouth, which I've never felt before in my entire life.

I thought it was one of the worst enemy of mine sneaked on me from behind, threw a gasoline bomb into my mouth. Innstantaneously, I became a blind although my eyes were wide open, and my eyes were profusely watery.

At the same time, I became a deaf. I could not hear any sound, although I cleaned my ear in shower in the morning.

I could not feel anything, although my nervous system was perfectly within normal range on my annual physical exam. My brain stopped funtioning, and nothing was going on inside of my brain. My mind went blank. I do not know how long time passed. As I recall, I was in a position that I looked like as if I was praying before a meal, as if I were a model Christian.

When I realized what happened, I gave a desperate warning to the people in my table.

And then, the moment I was going to stand up, and to make an public annoucement to the rest of the group not to eat any of the halopino if they picked up any of them, but I was a bit too late.

There was a sharp screaming coming from behind my table. It was from one of the lady who happens to be a soprano in her choir. When I turned around, I saw a lady laying down comfortablly on the floor with her arms and legs stretched pointing all four directions

Apparently, the lady took one bite out of the same kind of the halopino I had and passed out, and the soprano scream was not from the lady on the floor, it was from another lady sitting next to her, the victim of the same halopino that I had few minutes, or few seconds earlier. She was well attended by 3 well experienced physicians including myself from the group, and Ambulence crew came and gone empty handed.

As I mentioned earlier, Korean dinner table has more side dishes than any other country, which can be salty and spicy also, like the way main meals are cooked. This can be good for the tongue, bad for the stomach simultaneously.

For the best example for side dish, have you tried Kimchee before? Some Kimchees can be very hot, and can be very salty.

That is the reason why Korean foods are tastier and becoming ever more popular than any other country's food, because it is hot and salty.

I have to mention several of American, European foods also. People who like these foods are almost at addiction level not knowing how much salt in it, or they are madly in love with salt.

First one is bacon. A lot of people like this food, including myself, almost addicted. Especially, in the morning, if you are in a good hotel, you are being served with well-cooked, crispy bacon, and you notice that people go crazy. I'm one of them.

The other one is green olives. Olives itself is one of the best healthy food of all. But, I do not understand why It was made that salty.

It is human only who cooks food with fire, and puts all different ingredients to make the food taste better.

So the cooking becme part of people' or nation's culture among the countries.

Geopolitically Korea is located between China and Japan. Most likely Koreans took the advantage of both countries, particularly in food and cooking culture.

Go to the kitchen, and take a look at the cooking knife of each of these three countries, you can tell the differece immediately, and you will understand what I'm trying to say. Japanese cooking knife is slim and razor sharp. Chinese cooking knife is the opposite.

Korean cooking knife is just in between. Just take a look, you will see how differenrt cooking coming out of these 3 different looking cooking knife.

Aditionally, to make the food tastier, Korean food contains lots of garlics. Probably among those countries, Korean cooking probably puts more garlics than any other countries in the world.

This aspect, again, represents good and bad news to our body, specifically to our stomach.

The good news first. First, definitely garlic makes the taste better. Yes, much better.

Second, it can give us necessary natural defense against modern metabolic syndrome. Garlic is good for hypertension, diabetes, high cholesterol, etc. Garlic is also good against virus, especially against flu viruses. Garlic also gives us good immune system.

Even in flu epidemics all over in Asian countries, the flu virus cannot make any significant impact in Korean pennisula.

This is the bad news.

Garlic rich Korean food, or any garlic rich food, it has bad news for the stomach.

It is good for the tongue, and mouth, but bad for your stomach.

This combination of 3 musketeers, ie salt, hot pepper, and garlic will make our food tastier, and increase the quality of human life to the limit, but will make our stomach and the rest of gastrointestinal tract to pay the ultimate price.

Statistics and the truth tells us that the incidence of gastrointestinal diseases in Korean populations are one of the highest in the entire world.

I do not mean to say we should not eat garlic rich Kimchee at all.

But, we have to protect our stomach at all cost, with the cost that does not cost us much, with a minimum cost.

I am emphasizing that we have to consume those 3 elements moderately but, not excessively. If you eat too much of those three ingredients, you will end up facing potential problem in the future for sure. We have to keep the truth in mind when you eat these.

And take one Zantac a day for our stomach.

Second, the quantity, not quality, of the food we are eating in a meal at the table.

The large amount of the food can give a big headache to our stomach.

ADA(American Diabetic Association) advises people with diabetes to eat more frequently, which is smaller regular meal with snacks in between.

This is exactly opposite of animals, especially meat eating animals, ie cardavers.

When animals are not hungry, they do not eat. They eat only when they feel hungry. For example, the animals in the wildness such as tigers, lions, bears, and wolves, and so on, do not go out and hunt other animals for food, when they are not hungry. They hunt only when and because they are hungry.

Humans go out hunting for the pleasure of killing, Animals go out hunting only because they are hungry.

When tigers are not hungry, they do not hunt or kill, even when their best meal, ie wild rabbit is playing right in front of their nose. We, human, are the only creature who kills other animals for the pleasure of killing itself.

Let's focus on the amount meal we are eating.

In general, among humans, we can devide two group people, or cultures. There is one group of people, or culture, who mostly eat meats. A community thrived with hunting animals in the past.

And, there is another group of people, who mostly eat vegetables. A community main means of providing food on the table is by means of agriculture.

If we compare these two cultures, the apparent difference between the two is the amount, the quantity of each meal.

In meat eating culture, You do not have to eat a lot of meat untill your next meal, untill you get hungry.

But, in vegetable eating culture, you have to eat large amount of vegetables, and get hungry sooner or easier.

Now, the trend of meals are moving toawrd more meat eating pattern as the economy gets better. But, up untill a bit in the past, typical Korean dinner tables consist of a bowl of rice, usually big, at times huge, and soup, and 4,5 or more side dishes.

So, the ideal way of eating is to combine these two cultures together, and meet somewhere in the middle.

As you can imagine, if you had a big Mac with french fries and drinks, then compare to Korean meal or other vegetarian culture, Big Mac meals takes longer to get hungry untill dinner, it also means you do not have to have a big meal.

The stomah does not have a brain. So it does not think. It only respond to a certain stimuli. When the stomach is empty, it stays still, does not move. But, something comes in from the above, and the wall of stomach is being stretched out, that's the time they starts working.

The stomach mixes the food slowly, then moves the food down to the next station. At the same time, our stomach is producing many digestive enzymes along with acid. A strong acid that can give first degree, at times second degree burn to our skin. As a result of this, if the owner of the stomach happens to be a person who eat large, or huge amount of meals, it is inevitable for the stomach to get stressed out, eventually will end up with significant and/or serious problem, which requires medical attention.

As I discussed before, simply because we do not see it with our own eyes, it takes long, or longer, or untill it's too late, to realize, or recognize that there is some or serious problem going on in our stomach.

We need to protect our poor stomach from all different kinds of assaults, like salty food, spicy food, food with rich in garlic. and so on.

We have to keep in mind that a large amount of meal can make overwork the stomach, in the long run, there is more potential to hurt the stomach than smaller meal culture.

It was long, long time ago, when the tigers were smoking pipes. Actually it was about 50 or so ago, when I was in senior year in Medical School.

It was a time when the doctors had real hard time to treat Peptic Ulcer Disease, because there were not enough, or almost no medicines to treat this disease. Situation was similar in case of Diabetes.

Now, it is about PUD, then follows Diabetes next.

Not only it was time that there was not enough or almost no medicine to treat, bot also there was not a single diagnostic tool to make accurate diagnosis such as Upper Gastrointestinal Endoscopy as currently available and using.

So, in those days, if somebody complains of upper abdominal pain, or soreness, it was extremely difficult to differentiate PUD from other condition causing similar kind of pain in the similar location.

Then, in order to get some clue, where the pain is exactly coming from, the attending physician admits the patient to the hospital, and orders Upper Gastrointestinal Series, the only diagnostic tool radiologically, to be done the following morning,

This does not happen in the modern day medicine where everything will be done on outpatient basis.

So, the following morning, after the overnight fasting, the patient will be sent to Radiology department, where the patient will undergo UGI series. Series of X-rays are taken as suggested by the name, starting from Esophagus, Stomach, duodenum, and upper portion of small intestine after drinking a large cup of liquid contrast material. If you take X-Rays without contrast material, you cannot see anything.

This procedure, which I call the "Toture", not only to the Radiologist who performs the procedure, but also to the patient who has to go through the procedure. For both the patient and the Radiologist, the room that the procedure is being done has to be called "Toture Chamber." They will all agree with me 100%.

First, the Radiologist. Because he has to wear a gown, which contains thick layers of lead, covering almost entire body from neck to ankle to protect himself from X-ray exposure.

It is his lucky day if he picks up the responsible lesion in a several of trials, but if he does not, the torture for both patient and the doctor will last a lot longer.

As a result, many of my Radiologist colleagues suffers from low back problem, among those who end up having back surgery, ultimately being forced to have an early and unplanned retirement.

And, second, the patient. First thing in the next morning, the patient will be sent to the "Toture Chamber", where he will be confined untill the procedure is complete, and the radiologist says the patient can be released.

At the beginning of the procedure, the patient has to swallow thick white mucus-like liquid as many times as the "Toturer" tells him to do.

There is no mercy from this "Torturer" who continue to make the poor(?) patient to swallow this distasteful tasteless white liquid, untill he gets satisfactory result to his satisfaction.

Now, it is the attending physician's destiny, or decision, to treat the patient with something. But, with what???

The best weapon among medical treatment has to be diet, the porridge made out of rice. Actually, it is no salt, absolutely no salt, and no spicy at all, having no taste at all.

As far as I can remember, the one and only medication that is available to the doctor at that era was menthol smelling thick white liquid, called "Amphojel", which is basically the same as Maalox or Mylanta.

The nurse comes in, and give one teaspoonful of this white stuff 3 or 4 timed a day.

This is how we treat a patient who has, or who was suspected to have PUD.

In a modern day medicine, everything will be done on outpatient basis. The moment a patient complains of epigastric, or upper abdominal pain, depending on the urgency, either the patient wil be sent to ER for a emergency UGI Endoscopy, or be schedued to have elective UGI Endoscopy.

The moment the Gastroenterologist looks inside of our stomach, he makes the diagnosis right away, and comes up with the specific treatment plan, whether Surgical, or Medical.

If we decide to treat the patient medically, ie with medication, we have so many, extremely efficient medications available to us in modern medicine.

Zantac is one of those, which is the focus of our discussion at the end of this chapter.

Now, a bit about Diabetes.

About the same time, 40 or so years ago, it was not that difficult to make a diagnosis of Diabetes compared to PUD. But, the problem was the treatment of Diabetes, which was more difficult than PUD.

If you see a patient complaining of extremely and easily tired and fatigue, sudden weight loss or gain associated with 3 big "p" which are the typical clinical features of Diabetes.

Polyuria, a patient with Diabetes urinates a lot, and more frequently. Polydipsia, drinking water a lot. Polyphagia, eating a lot. You can make the diagnosis easily even before you do blood and urine test, which will confirm the diagnosis afterwards

Then, the headache starts. It is big headache of the doctors'.

Because there is not many medicines to treat, only a few but very expensive.

Third, the speed.

We have no reason to eat fast. But, if you look around, you will find many people eat fast, sometimes too fast. If you look at animals, most of them, or maybe all of them eat fast untill they reach a point where they do not need to eat anymore. It might be a good subject to have a research done why all the animals are eating fast.

Furthermore, it would be more interesting if someone does research on human nature regarding the difference between someone who eats fast and someone who eats slow.

We, human, unlike with animals, have no reason to eat fast. We control our own speed. And yet, among peoples, we can devide two group of people, people eat fast and people eat slow.

This is my question. Why some of us are eating so fast? Even though there is absolutely no reason to do that. Why? Why??

Sometimes, a person like me, who eats extremely slow, eat real fast when and if I have a reason to eat fast. But, the majority of the time, if there is no reason to hurry, I eat extremely slow, sometimes superslow, means too slow.

We can see there are two group of people, who eat fast, and slow, when we eat hard candies and ice cubes.

One group of people exhibit that the moment they drop a hard candy into their mouth, they break up the candy right away into million pieces with loud noise, and swollow it down. It takes only a few second for the candy to disappear from their mouth. Same thing happens with ice cube. Why do they have to break up an ice cube into million pieces. It takes only a few seconds also to disappear.

And, the second group. The people who eat a candy slow, may take forever to finish one 'stupid' candy. It stays in the mouth, and melts away microscopically, one molecule of the candy at a time. The same thing happens with ice cube also. The ice cube stays in these peoples' mouth forever, one water molecule at a time it goes down. And, finally it disaooears.

Ask yourself, where do you belong?

I hope all of you say you belong to the second group. Why????

Because I am concerned about your precious stomach. Why???

Then, which stomach will last longer and healthy between the two, fast eater or slow eater?

This is one of the big reason why I'm writing this book to help you to recognize the truth.

Definitely, the second group's stomach will last longer and healthy for sure. If you agree with me, it is never too late.

Please change and join the second group, that's where I belong, and live long and healthy all of us together.

So far, I have listed three main culprits that can impact our stomach nagatively. I would like to add few more, something that we are all aware of and then move to the conclusion of this chapter.

Unfortunately, there is something called "stress" that can hurt our stomach.

We are living under a lot of stress. Probably, under enormous amount of stresses. We are facing tremendously harsh competition than previous generation, and so on, nationally, internationally, socially, personally and at home. Stress is every where. We cannot hide. We cannot avoid.

I do not have to explain in detail, because we are all under so much stress, and always my stress, my hesdache is much bigger than yours.

Unfortunately, there is something called "cigarretts" that can give significant damage to our stomach.

Among us, we have friends who smoke, and cannot quit. It is one of my list of world's 7 wonders. Among us, there are many, who does not want to live long and healthy, and furthermore there are many who want to cut short our precious life. I'm wondering why.

Unfortunately, there is also something called "alcohol" that can hurt our stomach. Among us, we have friends, who drink excessively, and unable to control the impulse. This is one of my list of world's 7 wonders. I'm wondering why.

If we summerize all of these together. We, specifically our stomachs, are under attack by the enemies of our stomach:

(salty + spicy + garlic rich) food + large meal + fast eating habbit + stress + cigarrett + alcohol

In addition to these, we have one more important one is waiting for us. Probably the worst news of all the bad newses: It is aging.

Degenerative changes will make every single thing listed above worse, much worse.

This is the reason why we have to take Zantac, Guardian of Universe. No, it is Guardian of our Stomach. Take one before you go to bed.

Take one Aspirin in the morning, just before or after breakfast, or with a cup of milk. Take one Zantac, or Acid Reducer, before you go to bed, please.

Chapter VIII.

Black Madonna

There are numerous artistic expression depicting Maria, the Mother of God, typially the most famous one is "Pieta" created by Michaelangelo in St. Peter's Basilica of Vatican City.

Among those arts, some are expressed in color black. This "Black Madonna" has interesting reason why it is black.

From the biggest city of Spain, present and past, Barcellona, about an hour drive, we can visit, tall and dangerous looking rocky mountain called Montcerrat.

Usually, when you go to Spain in a group, the tour company schedule to visit this famous tourist attraction, "Black Madonna" on Sunday morning, and after lunch, then goes Gaudi House in Barcellona city in the afternoon. So, in order to digest this busy Sunday, you have to move fast.

To be able to attend the Sunday mass at 10AM, and listen and enjoy the worldly famous Boys Chior after the mass, you have to leave Hotel at 8AM.

By the time you arrive at the Church, I do not remember the exact time, Inside is already jam pact, the big Church has no empty seats, but standing room only.

After the choir, you have to go and stand in the long line to meet this famous "Black Madonna" on the top of the Church in a small chapel.

There is a good reason, why so many people want to meet this "Lady with Boy Jesus." Probably, this is the main reason why so many people come to this place to meet the "Lady."

In the early days of Christianty after the death of Jesus, St Mark came to Spain to spread the Good News.

When he finished his mission and retuned to Jerusalem, he gave this Black Madonna to the people of Spain. But, no one knows who was the sculptor. It is carved on the wood, the Mother sitting on the chair, the Son is standing in front of her, and giving blessings to the people. Her right hand is holding a tennis ball sized globe, and left hand is empty. But, this empty left hand is the one that gives us the miracles that we are praying.

When we hold this empty left hand and pray, the miracle will come to us whatever it may be.

But, this statue mysteriouly disappeared, and people forgot about the exisence of St Mark's gift of God's Love.

After hundreds years passed, it reappeared the same way when it disappeared.

When a young shepard was sleeping with his herds on the mountain, he noticed that a bright light is shining from a small cave.

He found the long missing wooden statue of "Black Madonna" in the cave, and brought to the village.

It was kept at the church of the village, but people of the village started noticing the power of the miracle that the statue shows.

In medieval time, when people pray in front the Statue for the safe return of young sons from a war abroad, or safe return of husbans from overseas expeditions, or sick member of families' speedy recovery, numerous miracles happened, more people came not only from nearby villages, but also as far from other neighboring European countries.

When Napoleon was in power, he decided to liberate Egypt from Turkish occupation.

On the way to Egypt, he was going to stop by this village.

The news that Napoleon was going to march past the village, spread out to the people of the village, especially amomog the leaders, whose headaches get bigger and bigger, also heavier and heavier, because what if Napoleon wants to see it, or Napoleon wants to borrow it, saying he wants to show the Black Madonna to his people back in Paris, or all over the France, and never returns it, then who will go and tell him to give it back.

But, if we refuse to give him, he will come and take it away by force anyway.

So, they came up with a brilliant idea.

They decided to hide the sculpture somewhere no one knows, and then tell everybody that somebody, like a thief, stole it away.

Indeed, Napoleon came, and send his men to see if he could see the statue himself.

They retuned to Napoleon with empty handed.

Again, time has come for the ststue to return to where it used to be.

But, there was one conern among the elderly, the leaders of the village.

What if Napoleon comes on the way back after hearing that the wooden statue came back to her place.

Or, what if another conquerer or strong figure comes to the village demanding to borrow(?) it for his own satisfaction, or for his own people's satisfaction.

So, they decide to make another statue, which is almost identical that no one could tell the differece.

Of course, the real one is hiding somewhere in the mountain in a cave, where nobody can see anymore. So, no one knows where the real one is.

In the beginning, as with real one, the color was wooden color, then gradually turn to black, like the real one.

Yes, since then, the one people are praying in front, is not real. It is fake one.

But, the very strange thing is that as people continued to pray to the fake one, miracle continued to occur.

For several hundreds years since then, how many people came to this wooden statue, and pray?

Astronomical? Yes, I'm sure it is more than the number of the stars in the sky.

So many people came and gone. Every one of them want to hold her left hand and pray. That's exactly what I did, too.

Again, she is protected by bullet-proof plastic panel like "Pieta" except her left hand, so that people can hold her hand while praying.

Before moving to next chapter, one thing I have to make it clear.

It is absolutely incorrect statement that many times when I said that people like myself, ie Catholics, pray to Holy Mother of Jesus.

Precisely speaking, we are praying to God the Almighty, no one else. And, we are asking her to tell Him what we need, or what we want.

I remember so well, that when I was little, if I want to have the same toy that my best friend has, then instead of asking directly to my dad, I convince my mom first, then my mom tells my dad what I want, then my dad never refuse or decline.

I learned that trick when I was very little.

That's exactly what we are doing.

Tell her first, and then she tells what we need to Him. Most of the time, he does not refuse.

We sound like we are praying to her, but the truth is we are praying to God, hoping He listen to this amazing Lady, and give us what we want, what we need.

Because we know, so well that the one who allow the miracle to us, is Him, not Her.

Even though I learn that trick when I was very little, I still do not know, or understand the reason why it works so well. I still do not understand the mechanism how.

To the best of my knowledge, I can think of two reasons.

First, He, the God, must be too busy to listen to my problem. God must be very busy taking care of other people who are suffering more than I am. There must be more desperate people in this world than I am. He is so busy and tied up with those people that He does not have enough time to listen my problem.

Second, He, the God, gave us "free will" as well as "consequences."

He is so fair.

If I choose to do something good, something good will happen to me. If I choose to do something bad intentionally or unintentionally, something bad will happen to me.

After I did something bad, and yet I want something good to happen to me, will He listen?

But, it is still a mystery to me.

Of course, we, the Catholics, pray to God directly, one on one, pleading, asking, and demanding, and so on. That's what I do many times. Why do I have to go through someone else? It's wasting my time and energy. I go directly to Him. Nothing happens.

Then, I pray to Jesus, His Son. Same thing! Nothing happens.

And, finally I ask Her to tell my problem, my difficulty to Him or his son.

How come He, or His Son listens to her??!!

I learned this trick long after I became a Catholic.

It took a long time to learn this trick.

First of all, I, myself, want to take care of my problem. If I took care of my problem, Why do I need help from others, including God. I do my best to solve my problem.

Second, if and when I have a problem that I cannot handle, I choose to talk to God, the Almighty, and the One and Only, directly, one on one.

If He does not respond, then I talk to His Son. His Son does not respond, either.

Both of them must be very busy.

Then I talk to Her. I receive the answer.

So, I have a big suggestion to everyone. It does not matter what religion you have.

When you have a problem, and need to talk to God, talk to Him first, then His Son. If there is no answer, go and talk to her, and ask her to tell either one of them, then wait and see what happens.

Here, this is the second half of "Hail Mary," my favorate. To me, in my opinion, the first half is not as important as the second half, although the entire "Hail Mary" is important.

It is as follows: the second half

"Holy Mary, Mother of God, pray for us sinners, now and at the hour of our death, Amen."

She is the one who pray to God for us to go the better place, and bury us in her heart.

How can He send our souls to a place where we do not want to go, such a place worse than the Heaven.

CHAPTER IX.

ASPIRIN

After I finished my residency training, I joined a group practice.

One morning, there was an old woman, who was admitted through Emergency Room because of a massive stroke, with paralysis on one side, I forgot which side was affected.

She has been seen by ER physician, and the duagnosis was well established by the clinical finding as well as CAT scan and lab results.

According to my judgement, her prognosis was so bad that I was planning to discharge within a few days, and called her daughter, and set up an appointment to discuss the long term plan.

But, about 3 days later, the patient showed a definite sign of improvement.

To me, I felt like I'm witnessing some kind of miracle. But, miracle did happen right in front of my eyes, which made me true believer of miracle of some kind.

5,6 days later, she was able to move her affected side with help of physical therapy, and began to speak.

After 10 days, by the time she was discharged, she was able to stand up and walking. Even though she was able to walk, she was discharged on a wheel chair, due to the hospital policy.

Before I discharged her, I had a lengthy talk to see if I can come up with a something that might be responsible for her alleged(?) miracle of sort.

Apparently, she had serious multiple medical problems, for which she was prescribed more than usual medications, among those of which there was one particular medicine that got my attention. It came out one of the over the counter medicines.

It was Aspirin.

Because she was suffering from a severe case of Degenerative Osteoarthritis, she was given and tried all kinds of NSAIDS(Non Steroidal Anti Inflammatory Drugs). But, nothing worked, and non of them were effective, except Aspirin.

Actually, Aspirin is at the bottom of the totempole among the family of NSAIDS, in terms of the effectiveness, especially for the pain control. Aspirin would be at the bottom of all medicines for pain control.

But, whether you believe it or not, Aspirin was the only medicine that works for her arthritic pain. And, she was taking rather unusual number of Aspirin pills a day. I do not remember the exact numder she was taking.

So, in my opinion, Aspirin is the one. Aspirin is the main reason she recovered from her massive stroke.

We, including myself, who have no reason to take Aspirin should take an Aspirin also. Even if a healthy person who does not have any medical indication what so ever, should take

Aspirin like this old lady, but not as much as, or as often as she was taking.

The reason is when we get older, our blood tend to become thicker for various reasons, that we have to thin the blood to some extent to prevent from thrombus formation inside of the blood vessels, particularly in the arterial side, thus to prevent the thrombus to become emboli to move from the original site to any of the distant organ, such as lung, brain, or heart to become the cause of pulmonary embolism, stroke, or heart attack, which are often fatal, or can cripple our range of activity, thus diminish our quality of life.

We can just take one Baby Aspirin only a day. One Baby Aspirin (81mg) is ¼ of an adult Aspirin.(325mg) I I recommend all of us to take one in the morning just before or after your breakfast. If you are too busy to have your breakfast, then drink a cup of milk.

Side effect is little to minimal, because you are taking such a low dose.

But, there are a group of people who should not take any Aspirin. For example, someone who is already taking one of the NSAIDS, especially who suffered from upper gastrointestinal bleeding after taking any of NSAIDS, someone who have blood dyscrasia such as leukemias or pernicious anemia, or thrombocytopenia(low platelet in the blood) etc.

Often times, many of my cardiologist colleagues tell me, that they advise their patient with heart problem to talke a handfull of Aspirin immediately, if and when they develop chest pains and/or shortness of breath before they call for an ambulence.

So, I, myself, wake up in the morning, before I start my day, I take one baby Aspirin, and go out.

Among those who take Aspirin already for one reason or other,

After a massive heart attack, he or she survives and is still alive, that is because she or he was taking Aspirin. If a person had a mild heart attack, that should have been a victim of massive heart attack, that is because, again, he or she was taking Aspirin.

After a massive stroke, he or she survives and is still alive, that's because she or he was taking Aspirin. If a person had a mild stroke, that should have been a victim massive stroke, that's because, again, he or she was taking Aspirin.

So, many people who take Aspirin, they don't know what Aspirin did to them, thus do not appreciate what Aspirin did to their body.

And, these are another examples of why Aspirin is being underappreciated, or being unappreciated at all.

There are many people like the following example among the stroke victim. It is literally impossible to collect the data, no one can give you numbers.

But, there were many researches done in a long term, double blind studies by national level in European conutries and America or by an organization like WHO, which showed statistically significant differences between those group who took Aspirin and placebo. Thus, it has been long time ago, since FDA approved to use Aspirin for the prevention of both Stroke and heart attack. We all know that we can buy Baby Aspirin on over the counter without Dr's prescription in drug stores. You have to make the decision to take this amzing miracle pill.

So, practically it is ongoing fact that there are many people, currently taking one Baby Aspirin a day, who are living healthy without being struck by a stroke or heart attack at this hour, would be and should be direct beneficiary of Aspirin effect

Often times, you might have heard about this kind of people among your relatives or close friends.

A victim of stroke, but never recognized by the patient, himself or herself, families or even caretakers. So mild that it comes and goes being never recognized. Sometimes, tongue feels numb, then the feeling comes back. And, back and forth. Sometimes, part of our visual field goes dark, and then comes back. And, back and forth. Sometimes, tip of the fingers or the toes goes numb, then the feelig comes back. And, back and forth. Sometimes, a person slips or drops her or his spoon or chopsticks for no reason. And, back and forth.

Often times, this is an early warning signal of oncoming a massive stroke. So, many of the massive stroke victims remember such epsodes after or if they survuve. We call this TIA ie Transient Ischemic Attack, aka Mini Stroke.

But, I'd like to call this Micro Stroke. Unable to see with naked eye, only able to see under the microscope. To me, "Micro" sounds more scientific than "Mini"

In such a condition of imminent danger of massive magnitude, it is Aspirin that will protect us by minimizing the result of strokes, from massive to mild, from mild to micro, from micro to nothing happened.

How wonderful is what Aspirin does to our body! What a silent hero!

Aspirin prevents stroke from happening in advance.

There are many people like the following examples among heart attack victims. But, it is literally impossible to collect the data, I cannot give you exactly how many. Simply, there are many.

Often times, you might have heard about this kind of people among your relatives or close friends.

Victim of a heart attack, but naver recognized by the patient, herself or himself, families or even caretakers.

So mild that It comes and goes being never recognized. Sometimes, it fees like real chest pain of heart, but sometimes not. Sometimes it is so mild that you ignore it. Sometimes you do not feel like chest pain of heart attack, you mix up with indigestion, gastritis, esophagitis, bronchitis, etc. So, up untill not too long ago, people thought and called "Acute Indigestion Syndrome" if someone dies suddenly with a massive heart attack at dinner table.

Many times, this is a kind of early warning sign of upcoming massive heart attack. Many of the victims of massive heart attack remember such episodes after or if they survive.

We call this kind of heart attack Silent MI(Myocardial Infarction), or Silent Heart Attack.

We may call this "Silent", but it will never be silent at all soon after.

In such a condition of iminent danger of massive heart attack, it is Aspirin that protect us by minimizing the result of heart attack, from massive to mild, from mild to silent, from silent to nothing happened.

How wonderful what Aspirin does to our body!! What a silent hero!

Initially, Aspirin was born to this world as one of antipyretic, and analgesic agent.

But, currently the FDA approved for more than few more indications other than initial purpose. There are many medicines that became more famous and popular because of "side effect" than the initial and original purpose of the medication itself.

2 best example: Viagra and Rogain

Both of them are developed initially for the treatment of hypertesion. Somehow, they turned out to have remarkable effectiveness for other conditions. Both of them made a fortune to their company.

Anyway, for the younger generations, they do not need to take Aspirin, but the older generations who start to exhibit the signs of degenerative changes externally, should and/or must take one Baby Aspirin a day.

Along with Zantac.

After all these explanation and evidences of why we should take Aspirin, if there is or are certain people that they don't have to or need to take Aspirin, how do we describe these people's behavior?

Self mutilating behavior, or suicidal ??

Once again, I strongly recommend to everybody except those who should not take Aspirin.

No matter how healthy a person is, if you are over 60 years old, you should take Aspirin.

81mg of baby aspirin is very tiny, so that it is so easy to swollow.

Simply because I strongly recommended Aspirin, I have not received any bribery, cash or any kind favor from Aspirin company. Not even a single penny.

It's same with Zantac, or Acid Reducer.

CHAPTER X.

"HEPBURN"

We have a very fond memory of two "Hepburn" who are not with us anymore.

We, ie the old generation, remember well Audrey (1929-1993), and Katherine (1909-2001)

We can see both of them at TCM (Turner Classic Movie) channel if we are lucky.

In this chapter, I'm going to talk about about Katherine.

I do not need to explain how good, or excellent she was as an actress, because I'm not in that business.

But, just the fact that, in the history of Academy award, she was nominated 12 times and received the best actress award 4 times tells us how good she was.

Although in the 21st century, a person whose name is Maryl Streep broke the world record of Academy award nomination with 13 times, but the winning record of 4 is still unbroken, and intact.

Every year by the end of February, there is Academy award ceremony. In early January, the Academy announces the nominees, then the entertainment world becomes noisy, and loudest on the night of the ceremony when the winners are announced.

This year, Leonardo Decaprio is one of the nominee of the best actot award.

He was nominated several times before, but never won before.

Always there was a darkhorse, who is not-so-good looking but with brilliant acting skill, takes away the award from Decaprio. There are more than several of so-called "hansome", and "good-looking" and, "commercially very successful", but never won Oscar leading actor at this time. You know who they are.

We have known him since he was little from TV, but ever since he became famous in the movie, "Titanic", I saw every movie he stared.

But, I was a bit concerned if he might be one of the many super stars, who finish their career without wining the biggest award in their field.

For example, in sports, such as Football, Baseball, Basketball, Ice Hockey, etc, especially in Golf.

There are many excellent professional Golfers, who made tons of money, but end their career without winning Majors. Once, there was a famous golfer, whose other name was "the best professional golfer who never won a major."

Anyway, unlike other actors or actresses in those years, many of whom become a movie star by accident, it was her childhood dream to persue acting career, and she majored in acting in college, then went to Holliwood to be a star.

Rarely, we see some people, not only who are very successful in their field, but also, at the same time help, and make others successful.

She is one of them.

She helped John Wayne, who never won a Academy, to win a Academy just before he died. I like John Wayne, not only he used to be my childhood hero, because I was growing up watching his Western movie back in Korea, also he invested all his hard earn money to his movie industry, he had little money left when he died.

And, she helped Henry fonda, also who never won a Academy, to win a Academy. He watched in a hospital bed his daughter accepting the award on behalf of her father. In the movie "On the Golden Pond, not only she helped him to win a Oscar, but also she took one for herself as well.

But, she has one big childhood psychological trauma. She was the one who found her younger brother dead, who hanged himself by mistake while practicing alone in the room a magic trick learned from his father.

The trauma must have been deep.

All through her life, she never put any make-up, except only when she was in front of a camera while making movies. She never wore expensive clothes, when she is not making movies, so that not many people recognized her if she is in the crowd. She never gave any interviews with a reporter or talkshow host with only one exception.

After she got married in 1928, and then divorced in 1941, she never married again.

And yet, we all remember that the famous relationship with Humpyrey Bogard, that they loved each other, but never got married.

The two became life long friiends each other while making the movie,"Woman of the Year," They remained as a friend to each other, untill he died of lung cancer. She took care of him untill the moment he died.

I visited Boston more than few times before to attend CME or other occasions.

But, few years ago, when I was making a schedule to go Boston again, I added 3 more days to the schedule to visit the state of Maine, up to the nothernmost part of America on that side next to Canada.

As soon as I arrived the Logan Airport, I rented a car.

First, I stopped by Cape Cod, and visited Martha's Vineyard, where John F. Kennedy used to spend his summer vacation with his family. Then, drive to north along the Atlantic coast line until I reach state of Maine, specifically to the Acadia National Park, which is my destination.

Then, turn around to south, but not same route, instead of going down Atlantic coast, change the direction a bit inland, to the direction of State of New Hampshire.

We visited Blue Mountain and White mountain.

Again, I realized that I'm not literary major. I'm a stubburn scientist, a doctor.

I cannot describe how beautiful, and magnificent Acardia National Park is. Blue Mountain and White Mountain as well. For example, when I went to Grand Cannyon, in front of the Grandness of God's magnificent creation, You feel the

Greatness at the bottom of your heart, not from your brain. How can I describe it from my tiny and limited brain? It is impossible. Simply, it's better to be honest, and give up.

You have to see it to believe it.

When you are under deep anesthesia by the nature, time flies.

Suddenly, you find yourself in the dark. Where did the sun disappear? You have to find a place to spend the night, and calm down your mumbling stomach. We found a small town in the middle of nowhere with help of GPS. We rushed to the town hoping that there is a decent resraurant.

Katherine Hepburn had a secretary, aka assistant, almost like her own sister almost spending their lifetime together. She goes everywhere her boss goes. They travel together if the boss has to go out of town or out of country for filming.

The secretary was given 2 weeks of summer vacation, that is when she goes back home, and spend the time with parents and sister and brothers together, because she travelled many of the places in and out of the country already with her boss.

So, when her secretary goes home for 2 weeks every summer, her boss also goes to the same town, but not together.

She rent a suite of the local hotel a little bit away from the town, and spend 2 weeks alone. Then goes back to New York, and continue her work as usual. She spends most of her time reading books in her suite, or walking on a trail. Occasionally, she appears in a local restaurant, and disappears quietly.

When I checked in the Hotel, suddenly the lady at the front desk asked me a question. Actually, it was an offer that I could not decline. How could I?

She said, "Do you want to have the suite, where Katherine Hepburn used to stay?" "There is no extra charge."

How can I refuse? How anyone can refuse?

I'm going to sleep in the same room, where she, the one I admire the most, used to sleep in the past.

I'm going to read a book in the room as she did long time ago, am I ?

Katherine Hepburn never gave any interview with a reporter, or any talk show host in her whole career, except one occasion, only once.

That was with Barbara Walters of ABC news.

At the end of her interview, Barbara Walters asked her one important question.

"Do you have Parkinson's ?"

We do not know since when, but she has been shaking(?) or nodding(?) her head continuously for more than several years. Because we do not, or cannot see her hands shaking, it is difficult to make the diagnosis 100%.

At that crucial moment, I was anticipating that she was going to say either "yes" or "I don't know" kind of response.

But, to my surprise, she did not disappoint anyone, including myself.

Her answer was very simple, it was just one ward.

"NO"

While she was looking at the interviewer eye to eye, she did not give any explanation whatsoever.

That is the reason why I continue to "RESPECT" her even now.

Chapter XI

Sleep

I do not need to explain too much about sleep. Because we are all expert about this issue one way or other, whether you are a good sleeper or a bad sleeper.

And, there is nothing much to add to what you know. We are experts about sleep, because we sleep every night. We spend many hours of sleep every day without missing every single day.

First of all, those people who do not have any problem in sleeping at night, do not have to read this chapter. Why waste time?

This chapter is written for those who have a serious problem in falling asleep, so called insomnia.

Like any other health issues, I'm going to mention how to solve the problem, and give you the answer at the end of this chapter. if you have problem in sleeping.

Anyway, whether you have problem in sleeping or not, we have to sleep, almost ¼ to 1/3 of our daily life, which means we spend ¼ or 1/3 of our entire life with our eyes closed.

Most recent study showed that 7 hours of sleep would be most ideal, but in my oponion, although I'm not expert in the area of sleep, 6 hours of sleeping should be more than enough.

Anyway, It is hard say one way or other, because everyone has different pattern of sleeping.

I'll do my best to describe about the insomnia, but one thing for sure is to tell the readers at the end of this chapter, the solution of insomnia, the answer to insomnia

I hope you agree, and choose to follow my advice.

In terms of pattern of sleep, there are 2 extreme, and everybody falls somewhere in between.

One extreme is that we know some people who go to bed, and fall asleep immediately, and then untill they wake up in the morning, they do not remember anything.

The only thing they remember is the fact that they went to bed the night before. They do not remember anything, even though thieves came into the house and cleaned up the entire house. I know several friends, couples, who go to bed, as soon as they finish the dinner at home.

Only a few exceptions for them to go to bed late would be when they have to attend wedding reception, some kind of dinner party, etc.

Yes, they are born to sleep, they are very happy, and they never regret the fact that they are in sleep more than 1/3, or a bit less than ½ of their lives doing nothing but sleeping.

What a waste, but these are a bunch of people, who are very happy, even though they do nothing but sleeping almost 10 hours a day.

And, the other extreme. I know only few of this kind of people compared to the first group. I'm very happy that I know only few of these people, only a few.

I'm introducing a small group of people who are on the other extreme.

These people are the kind of people who do not sleep at night, not even during the day.

I have seen a lot of patients suffering from insomnia.

But, this group of people are above and beyond the scope of insomnia. When they go to bed, their minds become more clear than before.

Even though they close eyes, their eyes are brighter than ever, so that they have to open their eyes. Staying in bed for 2, 3 hours without sleeping, it is becoming so painful physically and psychologically that falling asleep is ever more difficult. Then, here comes morning sun.

At the age of 60, this person does not remember that (s)he has had any sleep any night or day all his or her life.

This is a true story of one person's life, and I did not make up this story. And, it is also true that there are hundreds, thousands, millions of people in this world, who are suffering from so called 'insomnia, not worse than the person described above, but close to the person above.

I'm sure there will be a lot of people who are going tell herself, or himself that this is "my" story or "I'm" close.

So, I'm going to talk about the cause, and the seriousness of insomnia, more importantly the solution of insomnia at the conclusion of this chapter, as I always did, and will be doing when dealing with health issues.

Before I go into real, pathological insomnia, let me briefly mention about "artificial", or "iatrogenic", or "man made" insomnia.

I, myself, used to be one of those who had to go through this kind when I was young. I'm assuming there are a lot of people, who went through this "disease", and who are currently going through this problem.

I recall all those sleep-deprived faces including mine, who were preparing for the college entrance exam in Korea. Actually, the competition now must be much worse than when I was facing this challenge in the past.

And, more importantly, I always remember, and respect those people who work at night.

Especially, those are in the military who provide us, citizens of America, good night sleep. Also, those in the police, in the correction department, in the fire depatment, in the hospital, in the auto company, and so on, and so on.

They are the ones who do not have insomnia, but have to stay awake to protect, to provide better quality of life for the benefit of the rest of us.

I, myself, used to belong to this goup of people, so understand what they are going through.

We never forget thoese young ones who sacrifice to provide us good night sleep.

Now, I'm going to go over those people who suffer from lack of sleep, ie Insomnia, pathological lack of sleep. These are the sleep- deprived people who are so desperate and willing to take even narcotics to solve their problem.

It is relatively simple to explain the definition of insomnia. First, there are people, who have difficulty in falling asleep, who have hard time initiating sleep.

Second, there are people, who can fall asleep in the beginning, but wake up in the middle of sleeping. Then having hard time to go back to sleep.

There are many expert about insomnia, but keep their mouth shut or mull when it comes to the solution, ie the answer to this illness. The reason might be it is next to the impossible thing to find the solution for the insomnia.

Then, shall we go out, and find the solution for the insomnia together?

If someone does have a better solution than what we are about to find, let us know.

Not too long ago, in Seoul, South Korea, world renouned experts in insomnia gethered around, and had huge conference, ie symposium about "insomnia." And, they went home empty handed. Why? Even though I did not attend the meeting, I was not there, I know they went home without any solution.

If they found the solution, the entire world would be completely different by now. First and foremost, I would be completely different person.

I'm going to be happy and contented. I would be the most likable human being in the entire universe.

And there will be thousands and thousands of people, millions and millions of people like me in this universe, how can there be any disputes among the people, how can there be wars among the countries?

As a first step, why do we have difficulty in sleeping? What is the cause of insomnia?

And, furthermore, where did my insomnia come from?

You have to reflect on yourselves first to find what is the cause of your insomnia.

But, in general, let's find out what is the cause of insomnia. If we find the cause, then there is hope to find the solution, the answer for the insomnia.

At this point, someone can ask a question like this;

Why bother? Why do we waste our energy, while we have the solution already?

Don't you know we have something called "Sleeping Pill"? We can take one pill when we have problem to fall asleep. It's so simple! Wow!

Actually, the truth is there is no medication specifically manufactured for the purpose of sleeping aid.

Most of, if not all of the the sleep aid on the over-the-counter of any drug stores are one the antihistamines, which was manufactured for the treatment of allergies of our body, most commonly runny nose and itchy eyes. The major side effect of this group of medicine is drowsiness, and sleepines. There is no medicine specifically manufactured for the purpose of sleep per se.

And, the most commonly prescrobed medicine for sleeping aid is benzodiazepines, which is antianxiety agent, definitely not for sleeping.

There are short-acting, intermediate-acting, and long-acting benzodiazepines.

The most notoriously famous one, Valium, is one of long-acting benzodiazepine. And, the doctors are prescribing, and choosing one of those short-acting benzos.

These antianxiety agents are excellent medicine for anxiety, but it has addictive tendency if you like it. Yes, if you like it, it will like you, too. You cannot get away from it. It will not let you go anywhere. You have to stay with it, and it will stay with you.

That's exactly what happened to Michael Jackson and Prince.

The beauty(?), ie the nortoriety of these medicine is once you are addicted to the one of these, sooner or later your body will develop, or build up tolerance, ie resistance, your body demands more, and even stronger ones.

So, the medicine demands to increase the amount, more and more and more, eventually you have to change the medicine to stronger one. And, the vicious cycle ensues.

Initially, people start with mildest benzo with minimal amount, then amount goes up, followed by change to stronger one. Again, the amount goes up. And so on. This is exactly what happened to Michael Jackson and Prince.

You know the rest of the story.

When I go to Chicago, about 30 minutes before arrival, I pass tip of Indiana, a city called Gary.

That's the city where Michael Jackson was born. Whenever I pass Gary, Indiana, I think about him, and pray for him real quick.

When I go to California, sometimes I visit a city called Hollywood. If I take city tour with mini bus, it stops at many different places and the tour guide, usually the driver, explains what the place is famous for. The bus stops in front of or back of houses where a famous movie star, singer, professional asthlete, comedien used to live, or still is living, and explains about the house, and the person.

As one of the stops, the tour bus stops at a familiar(?) house, and the tour guide asks, "Do any of you know whose house this is?" Then, he explains,"This is Michael Jackson's house. He used to stay and live in this house when he comes to Hollywood. And, when he died, he went to the emergency room in an ambulence through that gate."

I remember the gate, althogh I do not know whether it is front or rear gate. I saw so many times on TV, so many days, and so many months, on and on and on.

I remember the house, and the gate.

In my opinion, he is the best, and the most talented entertainer of all time, one and only. There was no body like him before. There will be no body like him in the future in the history of mankind.

Sometimes, actually many times, I question God, the One and Only, if you gave Michael such a talent, and such a voice that only God can give, "Why did you give him insomnia and pain? Why?"

What is your message?

Among all of athletes, Michael Jordan would be the same. No one like him before, and after.

Somehow, both of the two who I like so much, have same first name. Is it coincidence or what?

Also, the doctors are prescribing anthistamine for sleep aid, actually you can buy it over-the counter. But, patients do not like antihistaminic sleep aid because antihistamine can give us drowsiness and dizziness after we awake. So, people prefer benzos.

Again, sleeping pills are not the solution for insomnia.

I do not know the mechanism of action of these medicine once it goes into our system, and how it is working on our brain cells. You can check Google if you want to know.

My main concern is; Whatever you take, or whatever you do, as long as we achieve the goal, which makes us fall asleep, I have no problem.

But, my concern is the addiction potential of these medicines. I do not want to be a slave of anyone or anything. I want to be free. I want to own myself, the owner of me, mysrlf. I do not want to be owned by something, or by someone other than me. DO YOU?

If you want to know what I'm talking about addiction potential of benzos, just look at Michael Jackson.

Once you become a slave of someone, or something, you have to do whatever they tell you to do.

There are many things like this, which has addiction potential such as;

Drug addiction, we are discussing mow.

Alcohol addiction

Nicotine addiction

Gambling addiction

Food addiction

I do not want to be addicted to none of the above. I want to be free. I do not want to be controlled by sombody or something other than me.

From now on, I'm going to discuss about the cause and the treatment of insomnia.

This is not something that I created by myself. It is the same with other health issues, the solution of and the answer of which all are what I learn from the textbook, in the classrom, and from others.

In my opinion, which I hope you all agree, this is the best and one and only way to solve the problem of insomnia.

If anyone has better idea, please share with me, and us.

This is the best and the most accurate explanation of the cause, and the treatment of insomnia, which is; very simple.

We have to be tired to have good sleep, both physically and psychologically.

Our body, our muscles has to be tired, and our brain has to be tired.

To put it the other way, if we are not tired on both, there is no good sleep.

I gave you the answer first, and then comes the cause. If we solve the problem of "being tired" or "being not tired", then the problem of insomnia will not be with us any longer.

To make a long story short, ths cause of insomnia is "being not tired", and the treatment of insomnia is "getting tired."

When I'm talking about "being tired", there are two aspects;

Being tired physically, and Being tired psychologically. These 2 things has to happen at the same time. If only one of the above is tired, and the other is not, then there will be no good sleep.

To give you the answer for being tired physically, there is one and only way to do it, which is exercise, which I explained in the chapter of "Exercise", the goal of this book.

If I come up with a formula, it is as follows.

Good night sleep = phycal fatigue + psychological fatigue

Does anyone have any better idea other than exercise? Please share with me, and us.

To explain about being tired psychologically, unfortunately it is psychiatrist's, psychologist's, minister's, priest's area, not mine. I mean they are better than I am.

When you are thinking about physical and psychplogical fatigue simultaneously, the good example of this phenomenon would be a young cadet in the West Point, or a young man or girl in the basic training camp, people like us going on a trip to Alaska, or Europe.

And, another talking point,

Insomnia is not a simple problem, much worse than common cold, or even high blood pressure, or sugar problem.

For those problems such as hypertension or diabetes, we have many ways to deal with problems listed above, either medicinal approach, or non-medicinal approach, or both

But, as far as insomnia is concerned, in my opinion, we have no other choice, but only non-medicinal approach alone.

We have, and there is no pill for insomnia.

You already know what that non-medicinal approach is, which is exercise. We cannot kill this monster with sleeping pill.

If you, whether you are a doctor or patient, think you can solve this problem by just taking a pill or two, you are making a big mistake. You have a big problem.

Especially, if you are a physician, and if you think you can solve this issue with a medicine, or a pill, think again.

Did your professor teach you that you can kill this monster with a pill? If your professor did not teach you, then it is you who create this monster.

Change your mind right now. Never too late.

Yes, we can kill this monster with short-, intermediate-, and long-acting benzos, and furthermore something stronger ones that Michael Jackson took, or was given.

But, look at the outcome.

But, once we kill this monster with pills, we are next. We get killed by these medicines, so called sleep aids.

Why do we go to the wrong road that's proven to be wrong?

In terms of medicinal approach, there is only one exception.

It is Melatonin. It is used only for the geriatric population. Young people do not need this medicine. The Pituitary gland in our brain produces Melatonin when the sun goes down. The darkness around us when the sun goes down stimulates the Pituitary glands to produce the hormone called Melatonin. That's why we feel sleepy becauce of this substance. So, melatonin is needed only those people who cannot produce enough to make us feel sleepy.

I do not mind elderly people trying this medicine. If it helps, continue to take it. If not, quit taking it.

This medicine, Melatonin, does not have addictive nature, which means it's safe to take, and safe to discontinue.

It is not my area of expertise, but something we have to think about. I'm not a psychiatrist, but we need to think about the insomnia as psychological perspective.

Many of the psychiatric illnesses do have insomnia as part of their symptoms, at times one of the precipitating factors of their illness. Only as a tip of iceberg, you will suffer from insomnia.

For example, 20 year old young man comes to ER escorted by 2 police officer because he was threatening to kill his family claiming that his family is poisonong his food. This is the first episode of his long history of schizophrenia, paranoid type.

But, his acute episodes always preceded by 2 or 3 nights in a raw of not sleeping, or unable to sleep.

20 year old young woman comes to psychiatrist's office escorted by the parents because their daughter locked herself in her room not eating or drinking, and not sleeping either. Her parents said whenever their daughter goes into her episode of her depression, she is not sleeping 2,3 nights in a raw.

Not only with significant psychiatric illnesses like the above examples but also with a little bit of emotional disturbances such as extremely angry or anxious or a bit of stress at work or home, we do not sleep.

Always we have to think deep, if we have problem with sleeping, to see whether this could be the tip of something serious down under or warning signal.

Sometimes, due to something called stress, we can have insomnia.

In any case of example listed above, we have to sit down, and spend some time to reflect on yourselves. I have to question myself, and ask "what could be the reason for my insomnia?"

If you think "it" requires to talk to someone, or expert, do not hesitate. You have to do it.

But, like anything else in life, you are the one who knows best what is your problem. Usually you are the one who can find the solution, the answer, the key to your problem.

Don't even think that a "pill" will make my insomnia go away.

If you are looking for the answer somewhere else other than yourself, you are one of millions who are looking for the answer at a wrong places.

So, when you think you have on going difficulty in decent sleeping, you have to look at what is giong on in your mind. At the same time, you have to look at the other side, and ask, "Am I working out enough?"

If you have a problem in sleeping, look at these two area. Please do not look at anywhere else. If you do, you know what will happen to you.

This is not a threatening from me. I have no reason to threaten you, my fellow human being. I'm telling you the truth.

Sleeping pill, aka sleep aid, is not something that helps you, or us to sleep well. It is acting like helping us initially, and make you feel so wonderful that you have found the solution for your problem, but sooner or later it will become our or your nightmare, easily will destroy us.

Sleep Aid becomes nightmare, and will make sure to be your nightmare

Yes, narcotic pain killer will make sure to kill your pain, and make sure you feel wonderful, and pain free, but sooner or later it will become your nightmare, easily will kill you.

Like the name, pain killers will kill our pain, but we are the next, it kills us.

Sleeping pills, and narcotics have strong addiction potentials. They help us to solve our difficulty acting as if a problem solver like a super hero, but sooner or later it becomes something bigger than me, something more important than I am within myself.

It is "pills" who decide my future, not me. What a tragedy! They make us lie and cheat our family, and our friends. They make us steal money, and ultimately make us kill other for not whole a lot of money.

But, we are the one who makes the decision. We make the choice, no one else.

When we were born, we were given free wills from God, the Almight. So, we are the one that makes all the choices. We are the one that make the choice with our free will. We get the credit if the result is good. But, if the result is bad, we blame God. We blame everything the God, if we do not get what we want.

I have a small question to my fellow physicians. Why we are not telling the truth about benzos, and narcotics to our beloved patients, so that they make right choices.

Both physicians and patients, we have to look deep inside of ourselves whether we are making right choices, not wrong decisions.

Now, let's turn to the general aspects of good sleep. Most of us already know.

We have to go to bed before midnight. Most ideal time go to bed is between 10 and 11. Never after 12.

Sleeping after midnight should not be a good one. Unless we have a good, and legimate reason to go to bed after midnight, go to bed before midnight.

Most recent research showed that 7 hours sleep is most ideal. So, go to bed at 11PM, and wake up at 6AM, most ideal.

Depending on the circumstances, it can be vary, but try to stick to the most ideal.

Just a little bit about taking a nap, aka ciesta.

There are some people who like to take a nap after lunch. There are some countries where napping is part of their culture.

But, first and most of all, you have to have good night sleep, and then take a nap. I do not recommend taking a nap after a bad night sleep.

There is a distinct difference between a napping and and sleeping during the day. What I mean is napping is not daytime sleeping. If someone believes napping and daytime sleeping is same, you have to think again.

First and foremost, when you are napping, 15 minutes is more than sufficient. If it is going over 30minutes, it is no longer napping, It goes into the range of sleeping.

I know someone who is taking a nap(?) every day after lunch at least 2 hours a day. This is sleeping, not napping.

What we need is napping, not sleeping.

Secondly, when we are napping, the depth of sleeping needs to go down to first stage of sleeping. We do not need to go down to the second, third, or fourth stage of sleeping.

When we are napping, we do not have to sleep. We just take a good rest with our eyes closed in a very comfortable postures, for 15 minutes or at most 30 minutes. Just close your eyes, that's all.

Proper napping will be an excellent medicine for our body, but daytime sleeping will be a bad poison to our body.

Because we do not need full 4 stages of sleep for napping. If we do, it will interfere our precious night time sleeping.

What we need to achieve from napping is rest, not sleeping. All we need from good napping is good rest.

HOW TO LOSE WEIGHT: THE ONE & ONLY, AND THE BEST

What???!!!

Losing weight? Are you sure?

Yea, indeed.

I'm telling you the best, and the one & only way to lose weight. There is no other way. Only my way. But, soon to be yours

If someone tells you there is any other way other than what I'm about to say, he or she is not telling you the truth. I did not say they are lying, but I said they are not telling the truth. This is why.

I'm writing this chapter in return for those people who spent their hard earn money as well as their precious time to read this "boring" book of mine. I'm sure this book is very boring, but many of you are going to have something in return.

For your precious time and money, I'm writing this chapter.

I'm going to tell you the truth for those who wants to lose weight. Whenever you are standing with the truth, you always win. That is the truth.

The truth that I'm about to tell you is not something that no one knows, but is something that everyone knows already. If any truth that no one knows is no longer truth anymore.

But, the truth I'm about to tell you is the truth that everyone knows already, but no one wants to tell you the truth the way it is, and no one wants to look at this truth the way it is, and face it the way it is, and overcome and win.

Who wants to come with me, and be the winner!!

The truth does not change, the fact does not change, they are always the same, but we are the one who have to change, not the truth, for the better based on the truth. Do not try to change or distort the truth, then ultimately you will be the one who suffer.

The moment you look at the truth, and make up your mind to face it, you are already achieved half way of your goal line. You are half winner already. All you have to do is to take an action, cross the finish line, and become a full and complete winner.

The only, small concern of mine regarding this truth, like any other truth, is that the road leading to this truth looks a bit narrower, and a bit harder compared to the wrong kind of false truth, which always looks wide open, nicer and easier.

Too many people have wasted their precious time and enormous amount of money while persuing the wrong truth, and failed to achieve the goal.

At the same time, so many of elite physicians, and scientists have devoted their valuable efforts to solve this problem, and failed.

How many times have we heared a news that some scientists found the solution for obesity, and then disappear from our memory like it never happened before.

Not too long ago, no sooner Opra Winfry came out in a commercial, and annouced that she lost about 28 pounds on a diet program of a certain diet company, than not only the sales figure went up sky high, but also the stock price of that company went up sky high too.

What a remarkable person she is.

But, if you are not standing with the truth, there will be a time to crash on the horizen. The truth is you can not solve the overweight issue with the diet program or system alone. How nice it would be if you can eliminate the overweight with one program or system. If someone is telling you that he or she can eliminate the overweight with diet only, or with one pill alone, that person is not telling you the truth.

Now, the truth!!

I'm going to tell you the truth of gaining and losing weight. This is the truth of the cause of weight gain and weight loss.

If you know the cause of a problem, you are already half way to solve the problem. Based on this truth, the cause of weight gain and the solution for the weight gain comes simultaneously.

It is the same thing, that the moment you understand the cause of insomnia, you realize the answer, the solution at the same time, by the same token, the moment we understand the cause of weight gain, we know the answer, the solution.

When you look at the truth the way it is, we are standing with the truth.

You have to keep this in mind all the time, while you are going through this simple truth. You have to keep this truth in mind all the time. Because, easy to remember, easy to forget. Easy come, easy go. If you think losing weight is easy, you'll never lose weight.

Let's think our body is a baloon.

When you blow a baloon, the more you blow, the baloon gets bigger. The air goes in, and does not come out. Where is the air that went inside? The simple answer is it stays inside.

Let's go back and think about human body.

When we eat the food, ultimatelly the food will turn into calorie that we use as our source of energy.

But, if we do not use the calorie generated by the food, where does it go? Where does it stay?

10 people went inside, 8 came out. Where is the 2? The truth is they are still inside.

It stays inside of our body as different form of energy source, such as glycogen in the muscle and the liver, as fat inside cells, and fat cell itself under our skin of our belly, etc.

10 people went inside, not only 10 came out, but also with 2 others, all together 12 came out, what happen inside. 2 person less inside.

This is the truth, nothing but the truth of weight loss.

If some one says there is other way other than this, that person is not telling you the truth.

Now, the 2 truth of gaining weight;

when & if you eat more than you spend, and when & if you spend less than you eat.

The energy will remain inside of our body in the form of fat as we all know. Of course, I'm talking about grown up, adult body.

Let's face the truth.

Here comes the 2 truth of losing weight;

When & if we eat less than we spend, and when & if we spend more than we eat.

In order to make it easier to understand, I'm going to ask a question before we go into any further.

What is the best and one & only way to spend (ie burn) the energy (ie calorie)? Many of you know the answer already.

Yes, it is exercise.

Exercise is the best way to kill, and eliminate fat cells. There is no other way, but to do exercise.

Again, this is how you gain weight;

If you eat more than you exercise, or if you exercise less than you eat. In other words, eat a lot, and spend (exercise) less, then you will gain weight.

Here comes the truth to lose weight;

If you exercise more than you eat, or if you eat less than you exercise. In other words, eat less, and exercise more, then you will lose weight. This is the best, one and only way to lose weight. There is no other way.

So, no matter how much more you eat, if you exercise more than you eat, you wii lose weight. No matter how much less you eat, if you exercise less than you eat, you will gain weight.

As you can see the solution based on the truth, is exercise.

But, I'm not saying it is not important to watch what you are eating. It is very important what you are eating in terms of quality and quantity of the food you are eating.

I'm emphasizing the importance of exercise, but that does not mean I'm ignoring the importance of what we are eating.

There are many companies and people advertizing their diet, their pill, their program, their surgery, their "system" etc. No matter how good they might be, if you do not combine with exercise, you are doomed to fail. That is the truth. You are going to fail.

If you want to lose weight for whatever the reason might be, such as Diabetes, Hypertension, Hypercholesterolemia, or Obesity itself, etc, you have to focus on the both end, what you eat and exercise as well.

I agree that it is an excellent program that Opra Winfrey 's advertisement.

But, if you choose to follow her commercial's program, or diet alone or anything without combining exercise, then you are destined to fail from the start, or even before you start, whatever you do.

So, this is my way, hopely yours too.

Eat what you want, watch what you eat, and exercise!!! Remember exercise.

You do not have to eat something that you do not like.

I do not need to talk about diet, or about what you eat in detail, because you know already about these things better than I do.

I do not need to talk about exercise in detail, because you already read about the exercise in the chaper of "Exercise".

Simply because it is difficult to face the truth, don't try to change or distort the truth. If you do that, the truth will become harder, and cost you more financially, not to mention about wasting your valuable time.

I mentioned earlier that we have two kinds of truth, one is changing on its own, or has to be changed with time, and the other is never changes no matter what happens.

Unfortunately, the truth of weight loss, and sleeping belong to the latter.

Before we finish this chapter, let's do a simple math.

Average calorie we eat a day is about 2200 k calorie.

If someone who is on average diet, is burning calorie of 2500 k calorie a day, he or she will lose weight.

But, the same person is burning only 2000 k cal or less, he or she will gain weight.

You cannot change this truth.

And, this is the result of latest research that I agree. Kind of a new knowledge and very interesting.

Something that we should keep in mind about obesity, weight loss, etc.

It is about tripple interrelationship among muscle cells, fat cells, and exercise.

It is possible to lose weight with diet only, but this research teaches us valuable lesson that shows us how bad the result would be when we did it with diet only, did not include exercise. It shows the ugly result of weight loss with diet only, without exercise.

I'm going to explain it to you as if it happened to a real person.

Let's say, there is a man, about 40 years old.

He, who likes to eat, starts gaining weight.

It has been known that when we are gaining weight, not only the size of fat cells increases, but also the number of fat cells increase.

That's what happens around our belly, butt, neck, face, and everywhere in our body. Our belly looks like pregnant woman, our neck becomes two, used to be one, and then our attractive double eyelid disappears one day without saying good bye.

One day, after shower he look at his body, and was shocked at the way he looked in the mirror.

He looked back, and regret what he has done so far. He realized that he ate too much stakes at the dinner, cheeseburger at lunch, breakfast at Coney Island, snacks in between meals like pizzas and chips with cola, etc.

So, he makes up his mind to lose weight.

He meets with a well known dietitien and gets a proven program.

He follows the program. He is very honest man, does not cheat.

After 6 months, 1 year and so on, he starts losing weight.

Finally, he succeeds to go back to the weight he used to be, his usual weight. He achieved his goal.

And, he is looking at the truth on the mirror again.

The truth is:

The person he is looking in the mirror is not the same person who he once was. The one he used to be, and the one in the mirror, does not look the same, and different. He looks similar, but not the same.

Let me explain.

This is the truth scientists found, not me.

When he gained his weight, as scientists said, the size and number of his fat cells increases.

Hypothetically, when someone is losing weight with diet only, without exercise, from where does our body draw energy that we need?

What is happening here? When we do not supply enough energy to our body, our body has to draw necessary energy from inside of our body.

In this circumstances, we, our body has two major energy reserviors. Of course, one is fat cells, and the other is muscle cells.

So, quite naturally, there will be 2 outcomes.

One is, when we lose weight with diet, our body attacks muscle cells to draw the energy to survive. So, the majority of weight loss comes from muscle cells.

The other is, when we lose weight with exercise, our body attacks and kills fat cells to survive. Quite naturally, the majority of weight loss comes from fat cells.

When someone loses weight with diet only, the one in the mirror looks like the thumbnail of when he or she was overweight.

His or her belly is still out, neck is still two, butt is still out, etc.

When someone loses weight with exercise, the one in the mirror looks like the one, she or he used to be. The person, he or she will be so happy to see her or his previous self.

Who will be happier person?

I hope you are the happier person in real life after you lost your weight.

So, the answer, and the truth is, when you want to lose weight, you have to exercise, at least you have to include, and combine exercise in your program, or your "system".

If you do not include exercise in your program or "system", it will inevitably fail from the beginning, or even before start, which I can guerantee.

To make it simple, ideal weight loss is; you have to do it simultaneously

Diet + Exercise, or Exercise + Diet

Please do not do it one alone, combine the two.

I hope you make a wise choice.

Chapter XII.

Isabella Stewart Gardner Museum

There is a museum in Boston, named Isabella Stewart Gardner Museum aka Fenway Court in the middle of the city.

The museum has lots of valueable, expensive, well-known, famous artworks.

I recommend very highly that many of you should visit this museum and see an artwork or more, "Oh no" not to see the artworks which is not there, so that you are paying your money to buy the ticket to see something which is not there.

I'm telling you the conclusion first, which is you are paying your money to see some artworks which is not there, to be exact, which was stolen in 1990, 27 some years ago.

There are not many people remembering this event now, even people living in Boston do not know and remember about this any longer.

Just looking at the name, it sounds like Spanish Queen's name, but she originally came from Ireland on father's side, and from England on mother side.

Both of her parents were born in very rich family. In those days, majority of immigrants were poor or very poor, but her parents were one of the few exception.

Isabella Stewart was born in 1840 in upper class of New York. She was the oldest of 4 siblings, but the younger ones died in young ages that she becomes the only one who inherits all of her parents' fortune.

She did not attent the publis school, or private school. Excellent teachers came to her house.

Between her age 16 and 18, she went to Paris for better education along with her parents, which tells how rich they are.

After she came back from Europe, she met her future husband, Jack Gardner, when she was visiting her friend, who also came to Paris for the same reason with her brother, and became friends.

They got married April of 1860. They had a son, who died at the age two with pneumonia. It is not uncommon that not only babies, or even adult died due to pneumonia because penicillin was yet to be invented and available. No matter how rich they might be, they could not buy penicillin.

Quite naturally, the rich couple makes a desperate effort to have another child.

But, each time she gets pregnant, the pregnancy ends up the natural abortion, aka, "habitual abortion" which means her femal organ cannot sustain the fetus through the full term.

Based on the medical science of 19th century, they had only one choice but to give up having another child.

When she was told there's no choice, shw fell into a severe depression.

With the doctor's advice, the couple decide to travel the world. At that time, commercial airline was not yet available, but they visited almost everywhere in the world. Of course, their favorite countris in Europe, Africa, Asia, etc.

Of course, they visited Egypt, and countries like Japan, Thailand, and so on.

That was how she was able to overcome her depression, by travelling.

The couple moved to Boston, and began their lives devoting, and contributing deeply to the city of Boston, including in art collection.

One of the local reporter wrote, "Mrs. Jack Gardner is one of rhe seven wonders of Boston. There is nobody like her in any city I this country."

In 1884, she travelled to Japan again, and China, Cambodia, and Egypt as well. She also visited England, and her interest and knowledge in art and art collection has gotton deeper and deeper.

In 1891, her father passed away, and she inherited all of her parent's fortune.

In 1898, her husband died suddenly of a stroke.

Since the death of her husband, she began to build a museum called Fenway court, and display all of her collections, while living on the top floor of the museum.

She develop and maintain relationship with artists and art collectors in Europe, and put much more efforts in art collection.

In 1919, December, she herself became hemiplegic after stroke, and die in July, 1924.

Before she died, she donated everything she owned to the city of Boston with one condition, which is, to keep everything exactly the way she displayed.

She did not want to look any of her art collection moved, or changed, or different from what she has done in Fenway Court, which is her baby.

But, In March of 1990, 95 years after she died, there was an accident(?) that her wishes, her dream has broken completely.

Ever since the museum changed the name from Fenway Court to Isabella Stewart Gardner Museum, it opens at 8AM in the morning and closes at 5PM all the employees go home including the Director of the museum, except 2 security guards untill the next morning.

At 5PM when everybody goes home, the security guards shut all of the museum's door, and do not open the door untill the next morning no matter what the reason might be. If somebody including the director, forgot something, then the person, who forget something, could complete the unfinished business the next day, although only the director had the authority to open the door afterhours.

However, while even the director was not aware of what was goinig on, something truly unthinkable happened on that night.

CNN had an one hour special report about this art theft 3-4 years ago, which I'm going to recall as much as I can.

It was around midnight of March 18, 1990, it was about time when, as routine, one of the 2 security guard was making round, while the other one was sitting on the front desk monitoring the entire facility, the door bell on the rear entrance rang,

Think about what is available now, and what not available over 25 years ago in terms of security equipment, or security system of 21 century of now and 20 century of then, there was tremendous difference.

Some equipments, which is everywhere and available now such as CCTV or GPS and so on, were still yet to be seen or available. We can only see the walkie-talkie, they were using for communication between the two, at children's toy store such as ToysRus.

By the way, motion detector was available, then.

So, when the security guard at the control center looked at the monitoring screen, he saw 2 uniformed Boston Police Officers at the rear door, asking or "demanding"(?) to open the door.

In stead of saying, "No", when he asked, "What is the reason?" why they needed or should get in.

One of the "disguised" thiefs yelled back and said that there was a urgent call from inside the museum and reported a significant disturbance that they had to get in and investigate what was going on inside.

The security guard in control center went into panic mode.

All of a sudden, in the middle of the night, like in Hamlet asking himself "To be?" or "Not to be?", this poor man stuck between the two question, "To open?" or "Not to open?"

Actually, he went into panic only thinking about "Should I open or not?"

But, out of the confusion, without having a chance to discuss about the matter with his partner, he goes into panic deeper and deeper.

Even though he had another two chances to get out of the situation easily, his brain stopped funtioning only to the question of "to open" or "not to open?"

Apparently, he had 2 choices which was very easy, both of the two are just one phone call away.

One is to call his director ar home, who will be in bed sleeping at home with his phone next to his bed, and then ask just one queation, "Should I open the door?"

And, the other one is call the precinct with which the museum had direct phone line. He can ask just one question, "Did you send two officers to us?"

When they came inside, they were pretending to look for something, or anything unusual while asking several questions to the security guard.

Then, suddenly, one of the "fake" policemen yelled at the security guard, and saying, "you look like exactly the murder suspect. The picture of you was posted on the wall today," then pulled out his gun, and, ordered the security guard to go to the wall, and turned around and face the wall.

As soon as he stood facing the wall, his hand was put on handcuff immediately.

By then, the other security guard came down from second floor. The moment he was asking what was going on to his partner, he was also handcuffed at the gunpoint.

They were taken down to the boiler room in the basement, and locked up untill they were found by the employee the next day after long search, because their mouths were taped with Duck Tape, not only they could not talk to each other, or scream for help to release him, or explain what happened.

According to the motion detector, it happened around midnight, there was no movement whatsoever untill 2AM, and then the action began.

They waited 2 hours without doing anything, while making sure everything on the right tract, as planned. And they disappeared around 5AM

They took 13 itens, of which total worth estimated 500 millions. Among the stolen items, "the Concert" which is one of Vermeer's painting alone is being estimated over 200 million.

Although I do admit that I'm not an expert in art, I value more the painting painted by Rembrandt, as known "the Storm on the Sea of Galilee."

But, why only 13 items? For two hours they occupied the entire museum. Why only 13?

This is one of the puzzle that FBI special units could not solve or explain the reason "Why" untill now.

First of all, there are more valuable artworks than those 2, but they did not take more valuables, "Why?"

And, "Why, only 13?" "Why not more?" They had enough time to take more than that.

If you go to the "Dutch Room" on the second floor, you are going to see the wall, where the 2 famous paintings were hanging, which has two big, gigantic frames hanging on the wall without paintings inside. They took those 2 paintings down on the floor, and cut it out with razor-sharp knife, and rolled the paintings, put the paintings insie of a paper cylinder, then they can carry as many art works as they can

You know the reason why, actually no one knows why, but you know the rest of the story.

So, when you go into the Dutch Room, and if you look at the wall carefully just above the fireplace, you will notice the two giant frame without paintings inside hanging on the wall.

If you stand in front of the wall, all you are seeing is the wall. Where you are supposed to see the paintings, you do not see the paintings, you only see the wall.

If you turn around and see the opposite side, you will see the self-portrait of young Rembrandt looking at you, or the wall, where one of his masterpiece was proudly hanging on the wall.

But, ironically no one seems paying attention to this empty exhibition, even though lots of people, young and old, female and female are coming in and then going out, without questioning why the wall is empty. Certainly, I could not find any notice exlpaining what happened or why the wall has frame only without paintings.

Although Rembrandt himself, to be exact, self-portrait of himself, must have seen exactly what happed on that night, he is silent. He does not say anything, although he saw everything.

I became so angry, and upset while watching the empty wall that I started mumblimg only I can hear," who did this? What a genious he is? What is his IQ?"

And, there was a group of people who seem to be having an field trip filled with fun and laughing, and gigling. But, they were very quiet and not disruptive of other people.

So, I talked to a lady who seems to be there's leader of the group, "Do you know the reason why the painting on the wall does not have paintings?" She said, "Oh, No." Then, immediately, "What? Did you say the painting on the wall does not have paintings? What do you mean by that?"

I told her that I could exlain the reason why very precisely, if she gave me an opportunity to tell the entire group, about 20 people altogether.

So, I spent 5 to 10 minutes of time to explain everything.

When I finished, everybody said at the same time, "Oh my God!!!"

Yes, indeed, It's "Oh, My God!!!"

I'm asking God to do something about this tragedy. This is tragedy to all of us.

For those who did it, and for those who cannot see it with our very own eyes.

Please help us God, move those heart who did it, and turn in those artworks to the lawful, and rightful owner, to the museum.

After 27 years, it is about time for the one or those who planned and succeeded, it is time again to do something right, "Return it."

You may not be able to return those artworks to the rear entrance door, because it is not existing anymore. It is demolished and disappeared.

You can return it through the front door.

If you think it is too much for you to return through the front door, then you have much easier way to do the right thing at last.

Return it to me.

You took it for free, you should return it for free. Do not feel sorry when you return, because you took it without paying, not even one single penny. It belong to the museum, ultimately to all of us. Let all of us, all of the humanity enjoy the magnificent production of one of our own humanity.

You know me. You know who I am if you read this book.

Chapter XIV

Alaska

You can travel Alaska in a group, or with a few.

For example, you can do it in a group with all of your families, your children and your grandchildren and so on.

You can do it with a few, in my case it is 2 couple, me, my wife, my best friend and his wife, aka Special Force of Travel Unit, like Navy Seals of the Navy.

Set the goal, research, and study, and attack the enemy, return home safe.

I do not mind which one you choose depending on your situation, but recommend "my way" with which you will get a better result in terms of spritual, or soulful journey.

Always remember, if you travel in a group, always there is one or two rotton apple in the basket.

The history of Alaska is rather short, but a bit interesting. When you are watching a professional sports game on a TV, if the team you are rooting for is winning the game, the game becomes more interesting.

When the Russian Empire and the premature stage of America were involved in a political game on the issue of Alaska, it appears the Russia was on the winning side.

At the time of the signing ceremony, at least Russia was thinking they are on the winning side.

Because, when the representatives of Russia and America went back their own country, they received the exactly opposite reception from their country.

Guess who received the enthusiastic, and who received the chilling reception?

The representative of America received the most chilling response you will ever think of.

Because he was blamed for purchasing a land with weather of winter cold in entire year and frozen most of the year, so that nothing grow from the ground, cannot raise farm animals, filled with dangerous animals,

In Moscow, there was a huge paty celebrating the huge success. They were whispering to each other's ear, "Those big nose Yankees, have no brain" for buying a waste land with such a big money.

In washington, there was a motion to fire the Secretary of the State in the Congress, for making such a lousy deal with Russia with an enormously high price.

As you you can tell, Alaska belonged to Russia, untill the time of the destiny, which was March 30, 1867, when the treaty was signed.

Quite naturally, in those days Russians were living in Alaska, not Americans. And, as a matter of fact, Russia needed Alaska to make fur coats, and fur hats, and so on.

The fur coat, and fur hat that Dr. Zivago or Shasha was wearing in the movie might have come from Alaska, made by Alaskan furry animals.

To catch furry animals, the Russian even came down to nothern California.

Russians were desperately needed animal fur to make fur coats, jackets, and mittens, and hats to warm up their bodies.

Initially, Russians themselves went out the wild, and catch the furry animals.

But, the job was not easy for Russians. To them, the Alaskan people, ie the Eskemos were far better than Russians, had far better skills than Russians.

Instead of venturing into Alaskan wildness risking their lives, they began to buy the furry animals captured by Alaskans with certain amount of money. But, the money was too precious that they did not want to pay for the furry animals.

So, they ask Russian government to send the troops to take the furs away froms the Eskemo at gunpoint. If the Eskemos refuse to go out and catch the animals, the troops take one of the families as hostage, and release the hostge if the young Eskemos bring enough furs.

Such an atrocity ended when tne Russians sold Alaska to America, and signed the treaty.

If you go around Alaska, occasionally you will be able to see small or large cemetary of the Russians, who lived in the area in the past.

What kind of a irony is that, when you died, you were buried in your country, and then all of a sudden, you are buried somebody else's land?

Probably, the Russians, especially among the leaders of the the country, for example, Mr. Putin, what will he think whenever he sees Alaska on the map that belongs to America since 1867, before 1867 it was the land of Russia.

Do you know how big Alaska is?

It is 1,717,856 square kilo meter, ie 663,268 square miles. If compared to Korea, North and South combined, is 219,155 square kilometer. It is 8 times the size of the entire Korean penninsula, just imagine it is almost 10 times of Korea, again North, and South combined.

It is bigger than Texas, also bigger than California.

For that, Russia received 7million 800thousand dollars, which means 2 cents per acre, and 4$ 74cents per square meter.

It was huge amount of money at that time, but let's think about current value of Alaska.

Can you imagine the current value of Alaska in dollars, the economic value of Alaska?

What about the strategic and the military value of Alaska? What about for the security of Canada and USA, have you ever thought about the value of Alaska, combing all of the above?

We can make a simple formula, which is very simple; especially strategically Something good for America, bad for Russia. Something bad for America, good for Russia.

Something good for Russia, bad for America. Something bad for Russia, good for America.

But, no matter how good or bad the deal was then, and is now, if you do not go and put your feet on the land, and move around Alaska, you will never realize that how bad to whom, and how good to whom.

And, another important thing we have to keep in mind, no matter how good, and how bad the deal was, and is, we cannot change once the deal was signed by both.

That is the reason why you have to think twice, no, more than dozen times when you sign your signature on the contract paper, not only it is personal contract, more importantly when it is between two contries.

You cannot turn back time. You cannot announce the contract is illegal.

Let's go back to traveling. We had enough talk about international politics.

Back to Alaska!

I mentioned before that it is better with a few of very close friends for Alaska traveling.

It was very helpful that my friend's wife have been to Alaska several times in the past, because her close relatives were living in Fairbanks, Alaska.

Big cruise ships depart from Seatle, or Vancouver, Canada, then sail north anong the coast line. I heard the cruise ship provide very excellent entertainment program.

But, I hope all of you, who travelled Alaska already, and who are planning to travel Alaska in near future, have some kind of spiritual journey or similar kind while, or after the Alaska visit.

This happened to be my spiritual(?) experience.

I hope all of you to have same experience like I had.

Yes, this is my way, and this is my opinion. Somebody can have different idea.

As I said more than once in this book, timing is important.

My window period of Travelling Alaska is from early July to late August. Unless you have to, I would not go to Alaska in June or before July, and in September or after August, which means I would go to Alaska only in July, only in August.

Take an airplane, and go to Anchorage, Alaska.

Those people living in Canada, or in nothern states in US, go to Alaska with their own RV (recreational vehicle) or rented RV.

It may take 7 to 8 hours of flight from Seoul, S. Korea to Anchorage, Alaska.

At the airport, you can rent a car that fits your own itinary and your personality.

It can be 4-door sedan, Suv, mini-van, up to RV. Unlike other airport, you can rent RV in Anchorage airport.

Then, you can go whereever you want to go.

You can go into Google if you need the direction. You need to look at the map once in a while. For the direction, you listen to the Google lady. Instesd of map.

So, from Anchorage, you go north in a very early morning, and arrive at coastal town, Weawold, where you hop on a ship to tour the glacier. It takes 8 hours for round trip of sightseeing.

The ship will stop by more than several places that you will remember long after your trip to Alaska. One of the sightseeings that you will remember is watching the humpback whales right in front of your own eyes. What a sight!

Then, to the glacier!

You are watching the glacier from the sea. I described to the best of my ability about the glacier in Canadian Rocky Mountain, where I was standing on the top of the glacier.

As you know I'm not a man of books, reading or writing neither of those two. I honestly confess to all of you, that it is impossible for me to write, or describe many things that I'm writing in this book.

This is one of the many. Glacier! Glacier! Glacier!

Instesd of describing it, I have to ask, dare to ask you questions that I can think of.

First," Glacier, Glacier, How old are you?"

Second, "Where did you get the color you have? Where did you get the wonderful color?"

Third, "How do you make the sound, What is the secret of the amazing sound you are making when you are falling to the sea?, Where did you get that voice? How is your vocal chord look like?"

Fourth, "Why are you falling down at this moment? Why now? Why are you trying to come close to me? How long did you wait for me? Why me? Who are you? And who am I ?!"

All I can tell you is this is the performance of the nature, created by someone upstairs.

But, among the performances, the most memorable moment is not the visual, it is the audio.

This way, I do not have to describe about the glacier and leaving up to you and your imagination. This way, I can avoid my responsibility to describe about the glacier. Now, it is up to you. You have to go.

But, this is one of the many moments of supernatural, spiritual, soulful experiences while travelling.

The only thing I feel sorry about the glacier is it is getting smaller, and smaller, shrinking and shrinking. It is going on even now, and getting faster and faster because of global warming.

There are many people, especially among the politicians, among the many leaders of one of the major political parties, and major religious groups, who do not believe, and even deny the what they are looking at. What kind hypocrite it is? Where did they come from?

I have no problem accepting the difference of opinions, none whatsoever! But, this one is fact. Why the many people say nothing is happening, when clearly something is happening right in front of their own eyes? Where are they from? Or, do they know, or see something I do not know, or see ? If so, let's share with us, and me, what you know or see.

The next day, in the early morning, I am heading to the Denali, the second tallest mountain in the world other than Hymalia.

It has been called Mt. Mckinley, named after William Mckinley, who was born and raised in Ohio, became the 25th President of US, assassinated in 1901, 6 months in to the second term, has nothing to do with Alaska.

Among the Alaskan indians, it has been called Mt. Denali, which means tall, high mountain.

From a distance, the native indians showed their respect and called the "tall" one. They wanted this "tall" to have their own name the "Denali. It was their dream to call the tall one tall

Finally, last year in summer of 2016, President Obama came to the park, few years before where I was standing and took pictures of my travelling partners and me with Denali behind, and had an official ceremony to call the Denali "The Denli, "officially for good, no more Mt. Mckinley. Mr. Obama did very good thing to the native Americans, and the "Tall" one, the Denali.

Dream did come true for the native American Indians.

Something about American Indians and Koreans.

Both of these two people originated from same place, meaning they had the same ancestors. Long, long time ago probably thousands years ago, they originated from Ural Altai Mountains in Central and East Asia, where Russia, China, Mongolia, and Kazakhastan come together, and migrated through upper China, and Southern Russia, then saperated in Manchuria.

Majority of the group came down to, and settled in Korean peninnsula, and continued and crossed the sea and went to Japan islands.

The other group continued, and crossed Bering strait, moved to the American continent, who became the native American Indians,

If you look at any American Indian and me standing next to each other, you will find many undeniable similarities between the two.

Before arrival, there is a small park and viewing area, where we stood and look at Denali, and a few years later, where Mr. Obama stood and look at Denali, and took pictures.

Among the tall mountain, with white snows on the top in the middle of the summer, and thick cloud around the shouler, there (s)he is, the tallest one, among the tall ones, standing taller than the rest, being called by the natives, now by the all Americans, you are the Denali.

Again, wake up in the early morning, go to the Denali National National Park.

Inside the park office, we find out, that we cannot go any further with our car. The parking lot is the finish line.

You have to take the park bus to go inside. There are many options, half day, full day, 8 hours tour. And, another option is, if you are a hiker, the bus will drop you off at a certain place, where you can camp, or spend the night at a cottage, and then pick you up the next day, at the same time, and same place.

You can plan ahead what to do at Denali National Park if you go in web site.

We took 8 hours tour with other tourists in a bus. The bus driver is also tour guide.

We have no idea how deep, and how high we are going inside. But, just imagine it is 4 hour of one way trip, some times the bus run pretty fast in a flat plains, and other times it slows down when it goes pretty dangerous steep hills.

On the way, and back, if you are lucky, you will see wild animals in the nature. we all know that we can see those animals at the nearby zoo, but it's entirely different feeling if you those animals in the nature.

You can see deer or moose, sometimes elkes and caribous when you driving remote mountainous area if you are lucky. Especially, elkes or caribou do not run away when we approach, although deers run away as soon as we make eye to eye contact.

So, when you see a elk or caribou, you can approach as close as you can, and exchange conversation with non-verval communication.

We saw bears on a two separate occasions, once in a group of family, and the other with one adult bear.

The park bus driver, also tour guide suddenly stopped the bus, and told us to look at a certain area of a creek in a distance. There was a family of four, one mama bear and three baby bears ware crossing the creek, then disappeared in the woods.

The second encounter was we were a bit lucky. Suddenly, the bus slowed down and stopped. The bus driver, also tour guide whispered to us to look right side of the bus.

There he is! An adult bear was almost next to us sitting in the bushes and small trees, and eating mountain berries picking up berries with his hands. He was so focused on minding his business that he did not care the bus stoped right next to him or not, he continued what he was doing.

Then, he stood up, and walked slowly to the opposite direction from us and disappeared. What an experience! It's like a "Close Encounter of third kind" in the nature. All of us had to say goodbye to his huge butt.

Another lucky encounter of wild animals in the nature.

This time it was mountain goats. When the bus stopped for a break at a place with a few small cottage-like builings and outside bathrooms. Not very far from us, we can see a rolling river, too. We were walkig around, and talking to each other how lucky we were, an so on. Somehow, there were 4 or 5 binoculars standing outside. The kind we can see in any metro or national parks, that we paid not much attention.

Again, the bus driver, and tour guide as well told us to look at the mountain slopes close to the top carefully, and see if we can find multiple white spots, slowly moving.

Indeed, there were many white spots in a group of almost 15 to 20 of them moving slowly in one direction.

When we told him what we were seeing, he told us to look at it with the binocular next to us.

Now, we can tell what those white spots are. We can tell the heads, trunks, and legs. Yes, they were moving. Moving slowly, but they were doing something while moving.

They were eating. They were eating grasses while moving. That's why they were slow. But, to me, although with the help of binoculars, I could not see any grasses.

Suddenly, something came to my mind out of no where. I asked the tour guide very interesting question.

"Why are they staying up there in the first place? To me, I cannot see any grasses up so high. I see only rocks, no grasses or trees up there."

Through the binocuar, I see only rocks where they are. Small and big, in all different sizes and shapes.

"If they come down here, I see a bunch of green grasses all around us. And a lot of water, too."

My tour guide kindly explained to me and others the reason why.

It is some kind of "Survival of the Fittness."

"When, and if they come down, it will be extremely lucky for them to have lots and lots of grasses everywhere. A lot of food, and water as well."

"But, there is one catch here. It would be always good to have enough food around them, but they can be excellent food for another hungry animal down here, mainly wolves, the preditors of the mountain goats."

"Yes, on a rare occasions, they do come down here, because they were too hungry, or too stupid. Sometimes we see the leftovers."

"Of course, some of the wolves, who are too hungry or too smart, go up the mountain to hunt for food. But, usually they are unsuccessful, most of the time they come back with empty hand, certainly empty stomachs."

"Because, on the ground level, the wolves run fast, certainly faster than the goats. It's no match. But, up in the mountain with rocky surface, the goats are faster than the wolves. Because their feet are well adjusted to that particular harsh environment. You know that the goats are excellent rock climers, don't you?"

Indeed, it is "Survival of the fittest."

When we are done with the Denali tour, the sun was about to go down.

We have to find a place to have nice dinner and decent hotel, or motel.

We found a good restraunt, and had nice dinner, but we got even luckier that we found an excellent motel, as it turned out to be later.

We were driving to the direction of Fairbanks, our next destination. In the middle of no where, we found one, with "vacancy" light on.

We went inside of the office, and ask for two rooms, then went to the room.

We found out that the room was a passenger compartment of a retired, old-fashioned train. They have done such an excellent job in insulation that once we turn on the heater, it turn into warm and cozy and very much romantic place. I was able to hear the wind blowing, the trees shivering, small animals playing each other under my room, and cry of wolves from a distance, and so on.

When the sun went down, and the darkness fell on us, though we are thrown into the Alaskan wilderness, I did not feel isolated or lonely at all. I felt like I was sleeping in my bed.

Then, we stopped by Fairbanks, drove to the north, and arrive at a small town Chene.

Too small that there are only a few traffic singals in the town. But, I saw a small airport almost in town, for the wealthy people with the private jets coming from everywhere, even from New York, etc.

Why?

For what?

Because, they have hot springs. It is outdoor. It is so hot, that you can see the steam going up from the hot spring. You cannot stay long near the hot water spring up. You have to keep some distance.

If you go to the hot spring after dinner, after dark, you can see all the stars filled in the sky, the Alaskan sky right in front of your nose.

It is so romantic!

CHAPTER XV

DENTAL HYGIENE

Gum disease and Hallitosis

First of all, this is not my area of expertize, so I have to be careful when I talk about someone else's issues.

Even though these 2 headaches are not only extremely important issues, but also by just talking about these issues, I can hurt the feelings of good people without achieving my goal. So, I put this chapter almost at the end of my book.

It is absolutely obsurd I'm talking about this, that there are so many experts aka Dentist around us who spent the golden years of their lives studying this science.

But, Dentists are reluctant group to tell their patients who have this problem, especially Hallitosis, which is their responsibility to discuss, and treat, but once you talk about this, there is high chance to lose your patients, they choose not to talk about this rather than losing their valuable(?) patients.

So, somebody has to speak up. And, that somebody happens to be me, who do not know too much about this important problem of ours.

Who will be the one who will put the alarm bell on the neck of a cat, oh no, on the neck of a tiger?

If not me, who is going to be the one!!

In fact, I had this problem also, and lived long long time untill recently I found the solution. The solution that I found happens to be so good, or so excellent that I want to share this with more people. Actually there are many people already who are practicing every day with excellent outcome.

As you know already, when I discuss about health issues, I always put the answer, ie the solution at the end of the chapter. And the solutions are not my own creation, or something that nobody knows. Actuallly, like the others, the solutions that I recommend are already known to most of the people.

So, the solution of Gum disease, and Halitosis are well known to the public. It is not my own creation.

When I talk to the people about this issues, approximately 2 out of ten are are using my method already.

This chapter is dedicated to 8 out of ten, those people who know about this magic but are not taking advantage of this magic.

I, also, learn this magic from one of my patients, and I shared this magic with my patients and friends before, and sharing this magic with you now.

If you are one of 8 out of 10, I hope you find this magic like I did, and keep for the rest of your life.

By the way, I forgot the name and the face of the patient, who passed his torch to me. But, I hope I do the same to you the way he did.

You can forget me, I give you the permission to forget me, but, hope you do not forget what I'm about tell you in this chapter.

Let me ask you a question before I talk about Dental hygiene.

Some of you know the answer already.

What is 3 most dirty pars of our body? I'll give you the clue, the 3, and try the list of the ranking from the worst.

This is random.

The opening at the end of the gastrointestinal tract.

The 2 opening, one on the right, one on the left, on the face just behind the both eyes, called ear canal. To be exact, external ear canals

And then, the mouth, that we are about discuss. Actually, inside of the mouth.

Depending on how you manage, the ranking can be different, generally speaking,

The worst, ear canal

The next worst, our mouth

Then, the cleaner than the other 2 ie the cleanest of the 3, is the opening at the end of the GIT.

Why ear canal is the worst?

The only way we can clean this area is with Q-tips without visualizing it. How do we know we are cleaning when we we think we are cleaning. Have you ever heard perforating ear drums while we are cleaning our ear canal, and then lose the ability of hearing?

I have seen, and witnessed so many victim of Q-tips. Even with Q-tips, how do you know you cleaned good? Did you see it? Have you seen your ear canal ever in your life?

Next, the mouth. We are brushing our teeth every day. But, brushing the teeth does not necessarily means cleaning the teeth, or our mouth. The mission is not yet accomplished. The explanation comes soon.

The opening at the end of our GIT, aka Anus. Many people take shower every day like we brush our teeth every day. We clean this area so good, because we think this area is the dirtiest of all, so that we make sure this area is crystal clean, so obsessively that we do not even have to look at it, because we are sure it is clean.

Is there anyone who checks his or her rear end on the mirror to see if it cleaned thoroughly. I do not. Actually, no one does. We don't need to. Because we know we cleaned this area real good.

However, we are going to start the mission to make our mouth the cleanest part of our body.

We do not have to explain that if we maintain our oral hygiene well or not, not only our quality of life, but also financial aspect of our life would be drastically different.

There is a saying, "Good Teeth, Long Life."

This not because we have a government issued statistics or a result of research from a big University's dental department. It is the wisdom of our life that comes from our elderly, from generation to generation.

However, it is those people, with serious dental problem, who believe this generational "wisdom" more than those with decent dental hygiene, little or no problem with their teeth.

Simply speaking, it is just a matter of time, if someone who has bad teeth, to mess up his or her stomach because the bad mouth ie poor dental hygiene cannot chew or grind the food properly and does not give well mixed food ready for digestion to stomach.

This means the dental health and the stomach has the same destiny, as the dental hygiene goes down, the stomah is destined to go down.

I do not know too much about Budism, but the Budda taught, "Life is the ocean of pain." which means our lives are filled with pain and hardship that we have to deal with.

Among those pain and hardship, one of the rare pleasure of our lives is the pleasure of food, and the pleasure of eating the food we like.

Whenever we eat, not to mention about the prerservation of species, we eat for the pleasure. So, to increase, and extend our pleasure by eating slow and longer.

I'm the happiest man on earth when I put a certain food that I like the most.

It's the same thing with the other one(?) also.

If someone is jealous about what I just said, I'll give you the answer, the solution to get rid of your jeoloisy right away.

I'm going to give you exactly how to get rid of Gum disease in your mouth. How nice it would be if you do not have this evil.

When you get rid of Gum disease with my recommendation, there is another evil one that disappears in your moth.

That evil one is called Hallitosis.

One evil goes away. Wow! One more evil goes away from my mouth as evil as or more than the first one. Wow!! Wow!!!!

Among the symptoms of psychiatric illnesses, the mind is so unstable that the patient sees something that is not there, hears voices or noises which is not there, and feels even though nobody or nothing is touching you. We call this unusual phenomenon Hallucination. (visual, auditory, and tactile.)

Does this mean that the foul odor coming out of our mouth so bad that we can have a hallucination? That's why we gave same first name? Hall---?

In Chinese language, they call the bad mouth smell "Evil Smell."

At this point, I'm going to leave it up to your imagination how bad it is literally.

It is up to your interpretation but it tells the problem we are talking about is very serious.

Anyway, It is not that easy to explain about the definition of hallitosis itself, but it is more difficult to talk to the people because there is vast area of misunderstanding about this problem. In other word, it is easy to hurt someone's feeling, the pride of someone.

This is so much sensitive issues that I would not recommend to discuss, or comment about this, even if no matter how close you are among your families, or your friends.

Just leave it up to them untill they find out the solution their own way, ans be patient, or

Leave this sensitive and difficult issue a person like me.

Hallitosis is the byproduct, or endproduct of the 2 evils, inflamation of the gums, and the decomposing foods stuck in between the teeth, which will not only damage our health with the smell itself, but also will give us bad influence in our interpersonal relationship.

For example,

Just imagine that leading movie star like Clark Gable or Leonardo Decaprio, whenever he opens his mouth, bad smelling comes out, what happen to the leading lady, who has to talk in a very close distance and has to kiss him many times throughout movie making.

Or, What if a physician, an internist, who has to perform a physical exmination all day extremely close to his patient, has bad smell coming from his mouth?

Or, What if, a genius, who just graduated Harvard, or MIT, and recently hired, was talking to the company's CEO in a close range about very important future project, or vice versa? The more important the project is, the distance between the two will be closer.

Or, What if a young man, who fell in love with a girl in his dream, is about to kiss her, his bad smell comes out of his mouth with nicotine flavor?

However, there is something we have to pay attention to, something we have to keep in mind.

The person, who has this problem, does not know or aware the fact that he or she has problem. My explanation for this phenomenon is we have a body that has super excellent ability to adjust to any environment we are under whether good or bad, easy or difficult, small or big, etc.

In this case, the olfactory nerve inside our nose has an excellent ability to adjust this environment, quit its funtion or numb itself.

No matter how bad or good the smell might be, if it is too strong, we do not feel the smell the way it is.

When we smell roses, if the fragrance is too strong, we feel the strong smell, but within a few seconds, we do not feel it as strong as it is.

This is why some or many are living with this problem long long time or all of their lives, without recognizing.

If someone knows that he or she has this problem, then the person is doing something or anything already, and successful already.

This is a true story, and real person.

In the past, in China, there was a national hero, whose name was Mao Tse Tung. As leader in his communist party, he unified China, which became the largest, and biggest nation in the history of all China. There was no Emperor, King, or General who achieved and unified the China as Mao did. There was no one like Mao in China's history, no one before, no one after in China's history.

When he became #1, the chairman of Communist Party, a dentist was asigned to him and his family. Later on, the dentist requested political asylum to US government, and lived in somewhere in the US. He wrote a book, his autobiography.

In his autobiography, he wrote a story of a person who had really bad smell from his mouth.

That person's name is Mao, the Chairman.

Probably, because he was too busy? If it's for that reason, I fully understand.

But, in reality, not only he has never come to his dentist, who only treated his family, but also never brushed his teeth in his entire life.

No matter how his personal dentist might threaten him, he has never come and seen his dentist.

So, as you can imagine, his fragrance(?) follows wherever he goes. When he sees his fellow citizens, or foreign dignitaries.

Once, he told his concerned dentist, pointing to the big Siberian tiger in the picture hanged on the giant wall, "Have you ever seen any tiger seeing the dentist?"

But, something that you have to keep in mind is, if any tiger overheard about this conversation, the tiger might say, "Even a tiger, we, living in the twenty first century, also see our dentist during our annual check up, like any people."

Even though we, human, have very excellent smell system as sensitive as any other animal, we are very generous to the smell coming from ourselves, which means no matter how bad my smell might be, it does not make me feel uncomfortable. But, it make us very uncomfortable if the bad smell comes from others.

Because of this rule of nature, similar smell from me does not bother me, but from others bothers me.

This strange phenomenon also occurs to the couples, too. When your bad smell and your partner's bad smell mixed together, and becomes our smell, it does not bother each other anymore.

When I was little, most of my fellow citizens (?) lost their teeth because of decayed tooth. We did not have good tooth brushes and tooth paste like we have now. We did not have Fluoride in the drinking water, either.

So, in the past, when we lost our tooth, the tooth looks ugly and dirty with part of the tooth missing.

Now, we do not lose our tooth because of decayed tooth anymore.

It is time now we lose our tooth not because the tooth itself, but because other reason, most of the time, Gum disease, scientifically speaking, Gingivitis. So, when we lose our tooth, usually our tooth looks every which way normal, sometimes in perfect shape.

When the tooth pulled out, the shape is intact, the color is pearly white, meaning in aperfect condition. But, they say goodbye to the owner with tears in its eyes. Actually, the tears are in the owner's, ie in our eyes.

Now, we lose our tooth due to the problem of surrounding structures, not the tooth itself.

Dentists were busy because of decayed tooth, now they are busier because of the Gum disease.

In the past, when dentist pull out, ie extract the tooth, especially if it is a molar teeth, the dentist is going to be in trouble, because it is so hard, literally they have to sweat it out profusely.

Now, it is so easy to pull out, because it is almost already out. Just pull it out. That's all.

In old days, when one or two teeth are out, then the dentists grind the adjacent teeth with no mercy at all, put something called "crown" on the top of it.

Now, instead of crown, dentists put, or screw in something called "implant". So, the adjacent teeth are saved from the no mercy.

But, whether it is crown or implant, a person like me has no idea what other peoples are going through, bacause I have no such experiences whatsoever in my entire life.

So, next, I'm going to dicuss why the perfect looking teeth are saying goodbye to the owner in tears.

I aleady gave the explanation that it is due to the failure of surrounding, supporting tissues including bones.

This time, I'm going to explain the reason for the failure of the surrounding tissue, at the same time, the solution, the answer to this problem, the prevention of the the problem.

Another good news,

When the Gum disease, ie Gingivitis, disappears, then the "Hallitosis" also disappears.

How nice it will be.

Our Teeth and Gum are well protected by our lips from the bad temrerature especially cold, from dryness, and excessive external force, etc.

Most of the time, our teeth are hiding behind the lips once it shows up, disappears immediately, like shy young girl, except only when we talk, yawning, or singing, etc.

Why is it such a hard task to keep our teeth, and gums clean? Even though we brush our teeth 3 times a day or more, and gargle with very expensive antiseptic solution AMAP(-many--)

Few month ago, I read in the news paper, and in the medical journal, that brushing the teeth can only clean inside of our mouth 25%, and the rest remains the same before and after.

I absolutely agree with this.

This is the reason why

3 most important causes of Gum Disease, and Hallitosis

First,

We have the most ideal environment in our mouth for the germs, bacterias, viruses, fungi, etc.

Like anywhere else in our body, our mouth is number one, if not, one of the best place that germs want to stay, and grow.

The mouth has the most appropriate temperture, and the moisture for the germs to grow. On the top of these two favorable condition, oxygen supply is blocked most of the time, but unlimited supply of O2 when we open up our mouth, meaning ideal place both for aerobic, and anaerobic organisms to grow.

No matter how cold, or hot outside it might be, inside of our mouth remains calm and peaceful.

In reality, our mouth is filled with all kinds of germs already, so if there is any kind of injuries in our mouth, the germ will grow like wild fire.

This wild fire will continue on day or night, whether we sleep or awake, untill it destroys completely the surrounding structure of our teeth.

Second,

We are injuring our mouth, specifically our gums all the time.

If you think eating food itself does not cause any injury to our gums, that's a big misunderstanding.

If you look under the microscpe, numerous injuries occur while eating, that's all the germs need, bacause germs are so tiny to invade into our skin, the barrier.

There are so many ways we injure our mouth.

There is one way to injure our mouth without thinking.

People living in cold climate, they have tendencies to eat or drink hot food. That kind of eating habit can give burn, first degree, or sometimes second degree, inside of our mouth. We do not have a good distribution of sensory nerve cells in our mouth, particularly in the gum that we do not feel that much of pain as we are supposed to.

There is another way. This is iatrogenic, and self-induced.

It is tooth pick. And detailed explantion comes soon.

Third, the most important,

The frame, the architecture of our teeth itself is the problem.

Our teeth itself, the structure itself, can be one of the root cause of our Gum disease. It is inevitable to have Gum disease. If we look at our teeth very closely, the more you look at close to the root, the tooth becomes slender.

Anatomically, the tooth looks like an athlete with wide shoulder with slender waist. They do not look like a fat guy with a belly wider than his shouler.

So, a little bit of different, but similar looking teeth of 14, sometimes 16 on the top and the bottom, altogether 28, or 32 teeth are arranged side by side, next to each other are sitting inside of our mouth.

So, quite naturally, there is no space between the shouler area, but plenty of spaces in the waist area.

Apparently, this space that I call, triangle of death or DMZ of death, simply the Triangle, or DMZ.

Below this Triangle, below the gum, the root of the tooth are planted into the bones of the Maxilla on the top, and the Mandible at the bottom.

In this Triangle of Death, when we eat any food, the particle of the food stick it in with ease, most of the times tiny and small in size, but occasionally big one.

And, whatever the reason is, when or if infection sets in, few of the abundant germ follows in, and our gum disease starts. Then, when the infection goes down, and down, and finally the bone gets infected, the normal looking, and the perfect shape of our tooth has to leave home sweet home, there is no choice.

Most of the time, the Triagle collects the well grinded minute food particles, but sometimes big piece of meat stuck in, try to take a small step to achieve the giant goal to destroy our valuable assect.

However, with good brushes and excellent toothpaste, we can clean the front and the back side of our tooth, and kill all(?) the germs inside of our mouth with powerful and expensive antiseptic liquids, there is no way we can reach in and clean this Triangle of Death as we want.

No matter how hard we might try, it is impossible to clean this area of death, and will be not much different before and after all the cleaning efforts you put in, and remember 25% only, that we are cleaning this area, except the method what I'm about to recommend, which we will achieve almost 100% of our goal to clean the Triangle of Death.

In other words, No matter how desperately we might brush our teeth and so on, and etc, we go to bed almost same condition without being able to clean the area where the cleaning is most and desperately needed.

You may feel fresh after brushing your teeth, that's all you achieved, feelig fresh. The dirty area you wanted to clean still remains dirty, or no change.

We need to change this! We need to add the thing I'm recommending.

In fact, even while we are cleaning, the Gum disease in the DMZ, the most, or the worst area we have to focus on, still continues to be the same at most, or gets worse.

Cleaing of this DMZ is the best way to iliminate the Gum Disease, aka Gingivitis, and Hallitosis as well, and the best way to achieve this goal, will soon come out, and reveal itself.

Before we get to the conclusion, I'd like to talk about a thing of very small, but also very important issue.

As we all know that not only all the teeth look not the same, but also their functions are not the same.

They all look different, and function different, unique appearance, and unique function of each tooth.

What I'm going to discuss here is about our canine teeth, especially the one on the top, on both sides, right and left.

Canine teeth? Do we need it? Yea, we need it for the cosmetic reason.

In the animal kingdom, for the preditors like tigers, lions, wolves, bears, it is vital to survive, to hunt other animals. They use canine teeth to kill other animals.

Why do we need canine? We do not need it for survival, unless you are a decendant of Count Dracula.

For the cosmetic reason, we need canine.

You will notice it immediately, if you see a person, who lost these two. There is a distinct difference between before, and after.

As a matter of fact, we do not realize it while we have it, but we recognize it immediately after we lost it.

Futhermore, people, your friends, may not recognize you in the crowd, when you lost your canines.

Have you ever seen a pulled canines? If not, any photos?

Among our teeth, it is the longest one. This root of canines stretches to, or passes the edge of of our nares.

It is so important, when it is in place, that it maintains, and supports better half of our face from being sunken, we look young and handsome in man, young and beautiful in woman.

I hope there is no one who believes that even after we pulled out such a big structure we would look as good as when we had it in place.

When the canines are gone, the area where the root of the canines were located, will go down "just a little bit", that we all are going to look like the face of the Wicked Witch of the West regardless you are a man or a woman.

To our most sensitive organ in our body, to our eyes, "just a little bit" makes a huge difference.

A person, who are old with age, with wrinkles all over the face, may look old, but maintains the way he looked when he was young, and people will recognize him easily.

But, a person, who lost both canines, no matter how many times he or she got botox injections, may look young without wrinkles on the face, but, even his best friends would not recognize, even if he passes by in a close distance.

So, no matter how old you may be, by keeping the face of your young age with help of your canines, when you happened to meet your old friend on the street, you can smile wide from ear to ear and become a competent old man, without covering your mouth with your hand.

If you do not want to cover your bottom half of your face, you have to keep your canines untill the day you die.

No matter how old you may be, if you want show your handsome face of your young age to your grandson, and granddaughter, and great grandson and great granddaughter, and so on, you have to keep your canines to the best of your ability.

Especially to all ladies, keep the fact in mind all the time, that keeping those two canines will be far superior to multiple botox injestions or face lift, etc.

This is not a threatening statement to justify the function of canines. Just ask your dentist. The answer is not very far.

One question.

How about an implant?

The answer is right there if you look at implant when it is ready to go inside of our mouth. Google it and look at the entire shape of the implant, especially on the part of the root.

It is not as long, or not as thick as real tooth. It does not replace the natural shape of our real Canines.

Let's go back to cleaning of the Triangle, DMZ.

What if we clean the area with toothpicks?

Apparently, using toothpock is the worst solution for this problem. Toothpick is one of the worst, if not the worst, enemy of our gum. The sharp front of the toothpick will poke, scratch, and cut our defenseless, innocent our gum at will, and introduce the safe house to the ever so happy multiple germs, because the toothpicks cannot see, they are blind, they do not know what is ahead, and they do not know what they are doing, which means they will do very nasty damage to our gum without any guilty feeling because they do not have brain, or heart.

If you want to or have to use toothpicks, then use it gently with extreme caution only on the front and back side of the teeth, never poke into the Trangle. That's when you injure your helpless and priceless gums.

Another question.

How about dental floss?

It is not as dangerous as toothpicks, but it is dangerous. Recent study showed there is not much difference between them. It is the same that they cannot see what they are doing. The floss can cut Tofu or hot dog with ease, as toothpick can cut through Tofu or hot dog.

Do you think your infected, deseased gum is stronger than tofu, or hot dog. I hope not.

If you floss the infected gum in the Triagle, the result would be the same or similar at best as tooth pick.

When you do it, as same as with toothpick, do it gently with extreme caution.

There is one thing you have to keep in mind.

When you use the floss, if you have to, make sure you are alone. Make sure no one is around you.

Not even in front of your family, or very close friends.

It wil be a big mistake that I can do it, because it is my spouse, my parents, my siblings, my relatives, or my close friends.

Apparently, They are the people who want to see your handsome, or beautiful face instesd of less than handsome, or less than beautiful face of you. The reason is, when you floss, your face turns from handsome to less than handsome, from beautiful to less than beautiful in a split seconds of time.

Not too long ago, in the Family Feud, one of my favorite game shows, there was an interesting question;

"What is somethings that a man should not do in front of wife or girlfriend?"

There were 7 answers on the Board, but I only remember 5 of them. I do not remember which one is #1, or which one is #7

This is what I remember: Do not fart. Do not burf at the dinner table. Do not curse. Do not put your pants down in front of her, and do not show your most valuable and, Do not floss after dinner. etc.

I was so glad that there are some people in this world who have the same opinion, or same feeling as I have.

Now, the conclusion, the answer to how to clean up the Triangle, The DMZ in our mouth.

It took a long time to come to this point, trying not to offend the feelings of good people.

To clean up the Triangle,

First, it has to be safe, so that it does not cause any damage to the gum to prevent the easy access for the nasty germs to cross the barrier.

Second, it has to be effective. It has to be proven effective.

I'm going to show how to fullfill these two conditions simultaneously.

Third,

The price. The price has to be reasonable.

With one condition: You have to continue what you are doing, what you have been doing. Continue what you do, do not stop.

I want you to add what I'm suggesting to what you are doing.

I'm going to introduce to you a small eqipment, that some of you already know and are using it already.

It is known to you Water Pick, or Water Floss.

But, the name of the product is Water Floss, and the name of the company is Water Pik.

Of course, you can find at any pharmacies, and Costco as well.

If something, or anything is available at Costco, I recommend Costco.

I explained the reason already, and you know that I did not receive anything from Costco.

A few months ago, I bought one for myself, because I needed a new one. The regular price was 79 dollars, but with manufacturer's rebate, I only paid 59 dollars.

Not many people are using it. If I talk to the people, about 2 out of 10 are currently using it. It rarely goes over 3.

I do not know who invented it, or what company did research and develop. But, I think it's worth to give Nobel prize. Probably, because it looks, and works like the "Water Gun(?)" in the dentist's chair, the Nobel Comitte decided not to award.

Actually, it copied the main function of the "Water Gun.(?)"

User's manual is in the box, but it is very simple and easy to use it.

The main machanism of the functionof this equipment is cleaning with forceful water. It cleans with forceful water like Dentist does with his "Water Gun(?). We can control and adjust the force, the velosity of the water If you run it with too much force, you can damage the gum.

This is the only one that requires caution.

I always adjust the speed of the water in the middle.

Naturally, the water temprature needs to be not too hot or cold, just warm is enough like our body temterature.

If you keep your mouth closed while you are using, the water will remain inside of your mouth.

You can do it before you go to bed.

Sometimes, some of the very smart people would mix a little bit of salt, or antiseptic liquid products to the water such as Listerine.

Before long, you will get your true smell of yours. It will come back to you.

Pretty soon, the gum disease, no longer, will bother you. And, the decomposing food particles disappeares from your DMZ, then the bad smell that bothers you and others that bothered you will say goodbye to you as long as you use this equipment.

And, the smell of your own body comes back.

When you wake up in the morning with your own smell, you will realize that I told you the truth, the best truth.

CHAPTER XVI

500

About one year to go for the Presidential election. it was Novenber of 1999, there was a small boat accident between the sea of Miami and Cuba, which nobody paid attention to.

Few people drowned, but most of them were rescued.

Nothing new, nothing surprising.

It was close to the beach of Miami. It was dark, but people in the boat were able to see the light on the building or in the street.

But, because of this small accident at the sea, almost at the beach of Miami, history of America has changed, which means the history of the entire world has changed as well.

The boat was too old and small to carry all the people on board, and started sinking

In the boat, there was a young woman with 7 year old son who wanted to join her family in Miami was one of the drowned. Because she gave to her son one life jacket given to her by the captain. And she herself swam, but she did not make it to the beach.

She wants to come to America, the land of opportunity like many others.

In this world, we all know that even if it is exactly the same action or behavior, the outcome, or consequences would be entirely different, or exactly opposite.

For example, if we kill a person in the street, we become a murderer. But, if we kill a person in a battle field, or many, you become a hero in your town, and your president will give you a special medal of honor.

It is not the same, but similar interpretation can occur in immigration issues.

Crossing the border either by the sea or by the land, the exactly same action will be treated entirely opposite way.

If you cross the border either by the sea or by the land from Mexico as a Mexican without legal paper, you will be treated as illegal alien. You will be locked up, and deported eventually.

If you cross the border, in this case most of the time by the sea, from Cuba as a Cuban, even though you have no legal paper whatsoever, you will be treated as a political asylum. And you will be given an American citizenship eventually.

Exactly the same action, and exactly the opposite outcome.

Not too long ago, when there was uprising against Chinese government in Tienanmun Square, there was uprising among the Chinese in the many city of America. Many of them went to Washington DC, and White House to demonstrate.

During this short time of uprising, Chinese were given the same right, or previlege as Cuban did. They can apply for the status of political asyllum.

So, in case of Cubans, they have to cross the sea, which is not a big deal in terms of the distance.

But, if they got caught in the sea, They are illegal, and will be doported.

If they step on the beach, evev though it is one step on the American soil, they will be given the status of political asylum, and gueranteed to become American citizen in the future.

It is real close between Cuba and Miami. In a good weather, You can see Cuba from Key West of Florida.

It could be close and very far at the same time.

It is close because you can see Cuba with your own eyes, and takes less than an hour in a speedy boat.

It could be very far, because you have to risk your life like this young boy's mom.

On November of 1999,

This young woman, raising a 7 year old boy, after being divorced, decides to move to America, join her family in Miami, Florida.

She escape Cuba with people who were in the similar situation, and with a same goal.

But, because of too many people on a small boat, or the boat was too old, the boat starts sinking, after they successfully avoided Cuban naval ship, and almost avoided US Coast Guard.

Miraculously, the boy was able to land on the beach, but the young mom did not make it to the beach.

The young boy, who lost his mom, begins his American dream under the care of his uncle's and his home, growing up with his cousins.

But, his American dream came to s screaching halt, when his father showed up out of nowhere, and claimed to have his son back to Cuba.

In the beginnig, it took the shape of a family feud that a father is looking for his long lost child.

Then, it becomes international legal disfute. Who has the legal custody?

The father wants to have his son back to his custody, and the boy's uncle refuses to send him back, stating it is boy's mother's wish to remain in America, and keep the dream alive.

So, it becomes a court case from Miami to Atlanta. And, finally even Fidel Castro becomes involved, who threatens to bring the case to international court, and humiliate the America internationally.

The court, also, leans toward the father, who has ultimate custody of the boy, his son.

The relatives of the boy, uncles and auntes, are becoming desperate as well.

Numerus Cubans in Miami are also on the side of the boy's uncles and auntes go out on the street, and in front of the court everyday.

Despite in this international tourmoil, the presidential election continues.

In the primary of each parties, Democrats elect the current vice-president Al Gore as their candidate, Republican Party elects a lot less known Texas Gonernor, son of former Psesident George w. Bush, George W. Bush.

When the year of presidential election, potential candidates anounce their intention as early possible, but most of them announce their candidacy early part of the year because of the primary election beginning in February, and March. But, by the time the primary election is over by the end of June, and each party nominates their candidate in their convention, we will know who is going to be the next president of United States of America.

In year 2000 presidential election, unless there is a major upset, or unexpected event, it is Al Gore, who will become the next president of the United Ststes.

Al Gore is Al Gore, current vice president, and the vice president of one of the most successful President in recent memory, Bill Clinton, except one scandal, in my opinion. The only disadvantage of Al Gore was the fact that previous 2 term of the pesident for 8 years was bt the Democratic, who was Bill Clinton.

George w. Bush, son of the former president, Georgr W. Bush. Actually, his younger brother, Jeff Bush, the current governor of Florida, is more famous, more known to be more presidential than his older brother, George. But, he becomes famous or gets notoriety that he did not allow or give any commutation to the death row inmate despite the plea from well known religious group, or people, even Pope of Vatican. Like a leader in the past, he becomes famous by killing people, and killing more people after he became the leader of the free world.

By the way, the election of the President of the USA is done by indirect voting system. It has been like that since the birth of America. The rests are direct voting system, Senators, Congressmen and women, Governors, Mayors, etc.

For the President, the citizens elect the electoral college of each State in November, who, then, elect the President in January.

The number of electoral college of each State is determined by the number of citizens, ie voters living in the State, ie the number of Congressman of the State.

So, the total number of the electoral college is; total number of Congressman of each State + 2(number of Sanators of each State X 50 State)

The State of California, which is the most heavily populated state, has 55 electoral college votes, and the State of Texas has 38, then New York, and Florida, each has 29 votes.

The exact number of electoral college votes varies just a little bit on each election depending on the population changes.

Accoding to the record, on the last election, the number of total electoral college votes was 538.

Any candidate who goes over half of the above number wins the election, and becomes the next President of United States.

Sometimes, not infrequently, a candidate who lost in total votes, but can win in electoral college votes. In some states, he or she wins the electoral college votes in a narrow margin, and in some other states, she or he loses in a wide margin. Then, the person who wins the election, but loses the Presidency.

The loser becomes the winner, and the winner becomes the loser.

That's the irony of the presidential election of USA.

But, it does not matter whether direct or indirect, who is the winner or the loser. Any election in any country or society, will be determined by the amount of money.

If someone says he can run a campaign and win a election without any money, the person is from the other planet, not from the earth.

In any society, or countries, whoever has more money or whichever party has more money, will win the election.

Particularly, in the American election you have to have money.

However, let's put aside money factor away.

Then, what is the next most important deciding factor in the American election.

Generally speaking, the candidate from the Republican Party has to win any election whatsoever, because of the above mentioned factor. No question about that.

But, the candidate from the Democratic Party has a good chance to win any election, also. What is the reason? How?

This is the second most, maybe the most, important deciding factor in American election. At least up untill now and quite some time in the near future, It will continue the trend quite a while.

Yes, the deciding votes in American election is, and has to be Black votes in my opinion.

Are you out of your mind? With only 10% of the entire population will decide the result?

Yes, when the Black voters come out, and vote, Democratic candidate wins. And if not, Republican candidate wins. Plain and simple.

If the Democratic candidate knows and master how to mobilize Black votes, he or she wins. If not, the answer is plain and simple. The Republican Party wins. That's why Republicans are trying desperately to make it extremely difficult for the Black people to come out and vote.

If you have any question or doubt about this reality, just go back to the previous presidential election up to President Reagan.

This is the truth, and the reality of American politics untill now and quite some time in the future.

In the general election, not to mention about in between election which shows far less participation than in general election, only more or less than half of us go out to vote, and a little bit more than half will decide who will be the next President of the US and the leader of the fre world.

That is the reason why the 10% of the black population is so important.

It is almost automatic that if they stay home, Republicans win, if they come out and vote, Democratics win.

If this formula stays the same, or does not change, it will remain the same pattern untill we see different pattern for a long time coming.

First, let's look at immediate past.

President Obama,

He had no problem to mobilize the black voters. On the top of that, he did not do anything negative against the whites and other minorities. But, on his second term, he almost lost the election after the first debate. His opponent's popularity went up so high after the first debate that he needed the help of Joe Biden, who saved him with the one and only vice presidential debate.

Even now, many Republicans are claiming they lost the game that they almost won, which I agree.

They were celebrating already even though 2 more debate remaining and long time left untill the election day.

As a matter of fact, I think Mr. Mitt Romney was, and still is the best Republican candidate who lost to Democratic candidate.

In danger of losing to Mr. Romney, who do you think saved Mr. Obama? Guess who?

Black votes and Mr. Joe Biden.

President Bush, the son,

Black voters did not come out and vote for the Democratic candidate. I do not even remember the name of Democrstic candidate, even though I voted for him.

Next, President Bill Clinton,

He is the genius of the geniuses, who mastered the truth of the 10%.

When he goes to Black community, or church, and meets people, he does no shake hands. He huggs everyone. It does not matter to him whether men or women, young or old, he huggs everyone.

That's why he defeated current President of US.

He is the one and only genius in politics. He turned around economy and avoided the desperate attempt to impeach him by the Republicans.

Only if he did not have Lewinski affairs, he would be one of the top 3, or for top 5 most famous past President of US history.

And, President Jimmie Carter,

Who is Mr. Nice Guy, Sunday School, Bible Study Teacher, from South, State of Georgia.

Unfortunately, He became one term president, because of Ronald Reagan. I'm going to talk about Mr. Reagan more on the chapterof "Heimlich manuever."

So, we elect our President, the leader of free world, with more or less than half of all the voters, and then, a little bit more, or sometimes less, when we have a strong independent candidate, than half of the voters will elect the President of USA.

Half of the half, ie one fourth, of the voters, citizens will elect, or decide who is going to be the next President.

This is the reality, the true face and the current address of American elections, which has to be changed one way or other.

It does not sound right to me, that the leader of the country is determined by the support of a little bit more, or sometimes less than 25% of all the voters.

Wake up America! We can do better than this. We have to do better than this. 25% of us elect our President, the leader of our country, and the leader of the free world. This does not make any sense to me. Does it make sense to you? Oh, no, not me.

Let's go back to the young boy.

In the court battle, it is leaning toward the father, legally, who has ultimate custody of the son.

So, the cubans, in Miami, and entire Florida, and the entire country, who support for the boy to remain in US, and continue American dream go out to the street, also start talking, and pleading to the politicians, Senators, Congressmen, Governor, and White House.

As the presidential election comes closer, they sit down and talk, and plead to Al Gore.

But, Al Gore himself, even though he is Vice President of US, and has very high chance to be the next President, cannot break the law of the land, and furthermore he, himself, has to follow the law, and reinforce the law.

Finally, Federal Court of Atlanta, Georgia decide in favor of the boy' father, and order to hand over the boy to his father.

The Cubans and the family refuse the verdict, and the tension grows between the two group, the law enforcement agency, ie the government, and the Cubans.

Finally, the law enforcement agency of the government, ie FBI, gives the ultimatum to the Cubans and the family and set the date to hand over the boy to FBI.

The family and Cubans knew that the FBI will take the boy by force when, and if they do not hand over. And, they organized a group of people like a body guard to protect the boy 24 hours.

But, on a hot summer night, heavily armed FBI agents surround and raided the house, and took the sleeping boy by force, gave him to the waiting father within a few hours.

But, everything was done like a lightening quick. In the middle of the night, when everybody was tired and asleep, a group of heavily armed FBI agents rushed in the house where the boy was sleeping, and took the boy away from the bodyguards at the gun point, and delivered the boy to his father even before the sunrise.

All the Cubans knew the next morning that the boy was long gone long time ago.

They, the angry Cubans, start swearing at the government, and ultimately at Al Gore, that they will not show up in November of that year or vote for Gore's opponent.

Yes, you guessed right, at Presidential election.

If this incident did not happen, or happened after November, we had Al Gore, not Bush as the next President of USA in that election.

The reason is, most of the Cubans are usually vote for Democratic candidate in presidential election.

They turned their back against Al Gore, either staying at home on election day or vote for his opponent, Mr. Bush, in retaliation.

But, not many people including myself, considered, or realized that this small event, ie incident will affect the outcome of the November election, especially Al Gore's camp, because major opinion polls showed Mr. Gore was way ahead of Mr. Bush.

So, the day of destiny came.

Presidential election in America always occur on the first Tuesday of November.

We are going through this interesting phenomenon everyday which is the sun rises in the east, and sets in the west, but on this particular November day we are not just going through it, we feel it to the deepest part of our skin.

Which is;

The sun rises from East, and goes down West. We have 3 different time zone in America, excluding Alaska, and Hawaii.

When people in New York, or Detroit wake up at 7AM in the morning, the people in Seattle, and LA are still fast asleep at 4AM.

At 9:30 AM, when New York stock market opens up, Dow Jones Industrials collapses and their retirement funds plummets to the bottom as in one Black Friday, the people in LA do not know anything about their fate, because they are still in bed sleeping like a baby.

When Detroit Tigers play in LA, the game starts at 7 or 7:30PM in local time, it is 10 or 10:30PM in Detroit. So, quite naturally, person like me has to stay up after midnight, or if the game goes into extra inning, I'm in trouble the following day, especially if the Tigers lose. Because I do not like my team to lose in ths first place, secondly, I only had a few hours of sleep.

Back to the election day,

People in east coast vote first, 3 hours earlier, and voting ends 3 hours earlier than the people in the west coast.

In reaity, while the people in the west coast are still voting, voting in the east coast are done and closed. And due to the advance in the computer system, the reults are coming out on the major news channel, while people in the west coast are still voting.

Sometimes, or theoretically we know the result even while people are still voting. Why?

Because, other than time zone, there is another factor.

Usually, but not all the time, those states on coastal area, east and west coast, are voting for the Democratis candidate, especially New York, New Jersey, Massachussetts, West Virginia, Florida, or California, Washington, Oregon etc, and those states in between go to the Republican candidate.

So, by the time we know about the result of New York, New Jersey, Massatussettes, South and North Carolina, Florida, and some swing states like Michigan, and Ohio, we can safely say who will be the next president of USA, even though the people in the west coast are still voting.

Many times, major medias announce the winner before the official result comes out, so called "presumptive" winner, by the time we know the result of Michigan and Ohio.

Almost all the time, the name of the presumptive and official winner do not change. I had to say "almost" because something happened the other way on that election.

Actually, on that election, NBC, one of the 3 major news medias announced that Al Gore was the winner around 10PM. Usually, about 10PM of the election evening we know the result, when the presumptive winner is announced, and it becomes official the next morning.

Of course, it was not official. It is presumptive. But certainly, I took it the way they said, the way I heard. I was not the only one, or one of the few who took it the way it was.

I went to bed around 10PM after I heard the presumptive winner's name, assuming that he, Al Gore, will be my president for the next 4 years, hopefully next 8 years.

But, the next morning, when I woke up and turned on the TV, news ankers are talking somewhat different.

There's is no official winner in the election. There is no official winner, because no one cross the magic number of 270 of Electoral College.

Because, there is no winner in Florida. They are still counting the votes. Actually they were recounting. And the number are coming out that George Bush is ahead.

Republicans are already celebrating.

Celebrating? Without the official annoucement?

By the time the recount about to be over, Mr. Bush is ahead by approximately 500 vote in Florida. Democrats are demanding to take the case to Supreme Courts, but the republicans were smiling, smiling big.

First, at the State level,

Who is the sitting Governor of Florida? The answer is Jeb Bush, who has same last name with George. Younger brother of George.

The most important question; Who is the Secretary of State of Florida? This time, her last name is not important. That person is a lady, and we do not need to know her last name. What is the most importannt at this juncture is what she is, not who she is.

This is what she is.

She is the one, as Secretary of State, who oversees and supervises the election process. And as long as her candidate is ahead, she will never change the number. She will never look at anywhere else. She will never make any decision going against her Party's candidate.

Then, the result goes to the Supreme Court.

Second, at Supreme Court;

The decision will be handed out by the 9 Supreme Court Judges, of whom 4 are on the Republican side, and 4 are on Democratic side. Then, who is the one? Who is the deciding vote?

He is the Chief Justice at that time, Antonin Scalia, who was nominated by Ronald Reagan, and confirmed by the Senate.

If the result comes from the Lower Court with Mr. Bush ahead, he will never vote against the Party that made him to be the Chief Justice.

So, it took more than a month the the Supreme Court handed down the decision that Mr. Bush is the winner of Florida's Electoral College vote, and as a result announced that Mr. Bush is the next President of USA.

Just before the Supreme Court came down the decision, while Mr. Bush was so happy to wait, Mr. Gore made his own personal announcement, which is definitely one of the best speech made by any politicians ever made for the sake of national unity, in front of fellow Democrats who urged Mr. Gore to fight untill the end, regardless of Supreme Court decision.

He said, "It's time for me to go."

As it turned out, this was the moment that the American history forever changed. And, the history of the world forever changed.

500 votes, has changed the history of America, and ultimately the history of the world.

And, you know the rest of the story. You know what happened in Iraq, and you know what happened to your retirement fund.

By the way, the young boy's name is Elian Gonzalez.

He is not a boy anymore, is a man now, older than 20.

CHAPTER XVII

HEIMLICH MANUEVER

When we eat, sometimes the food we just ate, got lost the right direction, can end up at the wrong area. As a result, the food, small or big sometimes, can block the air circulation to our entire body, especially to the brain. If such a dangerous codition last longer than 4 to 6 minutes, it will leave permanent brain damage, ultimately result in death if oxygen supply remain shut down.

In such an iminent danger of life or death, there is a manuever availale that makes to turn our lives from death to a new life.

What is it? What is that giving us a new life?

It is written above: Heimlich manuever.

Henry Heimlich, M.D., the creator of this manuever, was born in the city of Willmington, Delaware, on Feb 3, 1920. He is living in Cincinati, Ohio. Still very healthy.

In 1974, he introduced this manuever for the first time through American Heart Association.

Ever since, this manuever has been spread out to the entire world, and we do not know how many peoples' lives have been saved, because we do not have official data for this particular area.

We do not know how many people have been given a new life.

He should have been awarded Nobel Prize long time ago, but there no official report yet.

Anyway,

Before Heimlich manuever was introduced, when a piece of food block the airway, people used to blow hard on the back of the victim with palm of the hand over and over. We call this Back Blow method.

Currently, American Red Cross recommends, and teaches first responders and medical professionals to attemt Back Blow method twice or three times, then to attempt Heimlich manuever if Back Blow is unsuccessful.

So, the disfute, and conflict between American Red Cross and Dr. Heimlich still continues, because American Red Cross insists to attempt Back Blow first, followed by Heimlich manuever, and Dr. Heimlich continues to preach to attempt Heimlich manuever first.

According to Dr. Heimlich, if we blow hard the back of choking victim, due to the pain and loud noise, it is human nature ie physiological response, ie reflex of our body to inhale, which will create negative pressure in our chest cavity, which will make the foreign body go down further.

And, the disfute continues, but neither side is going to prevail.

The reason is;

We can not perform a research about which method is superior to the other. Maybe we can go up to the animal study. But, we cannot experiment this to human being.

248

There will be no human volunteers for this research, no, absolutely not. Who will volunteer for this? At what price? You? Or me? No, not you, or not me.

So the dispute continues. No one knows when it will end.

But, you will find out which side I am standing if, and when you finish reading this chapter. You will get the answer if you continue to read.

It is up to you which method you apply, and which side you are standing.

What is important is you have to save a choking person. It does not matter which method you apply. You have no time to think which one you are going to choose. Not even one second for this, because one second might make the difference between life or the other. You know what I mean.

The core content of the Heimlich manuever is abdominal thrust. Unfortunitely we call a person choking victim, who is on tne crossroad of life or death due to foreign body, usually food, stuck in the airway.

Instantaneously and aggressively, we put strong pressure on the middle portion between the belly button and the lower portion of the sternum.

Most common position is like a bear hugs a tree, we(I) position ourselves(myself) back of a choking victim. And then, put sudden pressure toward me as if I'm having a convulsion.

If the choking victim happens to be too big for me to grab from behind, I can put the person on the hard floor, and go on the top of the person, with both hands together, then do the same.

In case of children, the performer sits down on the chair, put the victim on the lap and do the same.

When you hold your hand together, put your stronger hand, righties right hand, lefties left hand, 90 degrees toward the victim. Thumb and index side toward the victim which will deliver the maximum blow, not the palm side which is flat, which wil not give the maximum blow.

In a peaceful moment, when you go to a good restraunt with your family, or friends, having a quality time, a person next to your table suddenly became a choking victim.

When a piece of meat enters to the wrong way and blocks airway, usually the person does his best to remove it, and then, if unsuccessful, will make strange noise and then grab his or her neck with both hands and tries to stand up but unable to do it. That is when the person next to the victm recognizes what happened.

The person will witness the typical posture of choking victim, with both hands grabbing his or her neck, and face turn blue, or dark blue, even black.

This is the moment of truth. At this crucial moment, somebody or anybody nearby, calmly goes around the victim's back, and performs Heimlich manuever.

I guerantee you the color of the victim's comes back to normal, and the person wil talk again, saying, "Thank you, Thank you, Thank you." He or she will begin his or her life thanking for everything every day for the rest of his or her life.

This is not what I said. Dr. Heimlich said.

But, at this crucial moment, if everybody becomes panicky and confused, you know the rest of the story. Even if ambulence and first responders show up, after 4 to 6 minutes, the story ends.

However, if you count calmly, "one, and two and three....." and so on, do what you have to do one at a time, 4 to 6 minutes is not so short, is not going to be that short as you might think. It is long enough to save a person's life. But if you are in panic, and not doing what you are supposed to do, like anything else, the time flies.

It is as simple as that.

Again, and again, calmly step to the back of the victim, and perform Heimlich manuever.

Calm outside, even though panicky inside.

Even though in the book, they advise up to 5 times and think about next step, or something else. However, you have to do more than 5 times if necessary.

American Red Cross advises 5 times of Back Blow, followed by 5 times of Heimlich manuever.

And then, we have to decide whether we have to go to the next step, if Heimlich manuever does not solve the problem.

In case we fail to bring up the blocking foreign body, the story does not end at that point.

The moment we move to next step after 5 or more attempts of Heimlich manuever, the purpose changes, from the removal of foreign body to saving human life, which is the ultimate goal of every thing we do.

We have to move to CPR.(CardioPulmonary Resuscitation)

As soon as you made the decision to do CPR, you tell the person next to you to call Ambulence. And then, you start CPR, one man or two men, untill the First Responder arrive.

So far, it was the example of the choking victim, and about what you can do.

But, if you happened to see a unconscious person in the dark corner of a street, you have shake the person first to see if the person is sleeping, or unconscious, if unconscious, tell the bystandes to call an Ambulence, and start CPR immediately.

But, one thing clear.

No matter what the outcome might have been, even if the result is negative, the performer is not responsible for the bad outcome.

Successful or not, the performer is not responsible. The performer is protected by the law, which is Good Samaritan Law.

Do not worry about bad outcome. It is not your fault. It is victim's fault for the bad luck.

Back to the story of mine.

I jump into a society with which I have little knowledge, and absolutely no experience at all. It is like jumping into Pacific Ocean for a person who never learn swimming.

All I had was the fact that I was young and had blind courage. I was afraid of nothing. I had no doubt in my mind that I will succeed in my life. But, I did not have a slightest idea that life is not easy, and this much difficult.

At the time I came to America, Ronald Reagan was the president. Somebody who failed as an actor, and as a husband. But, he was very much successful as a politician.

Someone who beat up the current president, then became newly elected president.

It appears calm outside, but internally turmoil brewing real hard. Unexpectedly, suddenly political environment changed from Jimmy Carter to Ronald Reagan, from Democratc President to Republican President, from Socialism to Capitalism. America need sufficient time to change. It is too short for entire country to change from one philosophy to another. 4 years is too short.

It is like Pacific Ocean, peaceful superfially, but turbulence brewing at the bottom.

The enormous change that Mr. Reagan was about to bring to the entire country is about to start.

Particularly, after First and Second World War, the entire county was suffering from high unemployment and deepened poverty for a lot of soldiers released from military forces looking for job.

To solve these serious and significant national issues, naturally Democratic Party's socialistic approach attracts majority of people's mind as more viable solution.

Now the government becomes the center of the solution and the problem simutaneously. The government becomes the leader fightng the ever-growing poverty and biggest employee. One after another, government makes big announcement of enormous projects, which employs young poor, and unemployed, was pouring out to the society from military.

Mr. Reagan becomes a rising star in Republican Party, pointing out government beaurocracy, and, wherever he goes, he lays out his agenda, his solution. He emphasizes,"Small but efficient Government. And yet, strong military."

A lot of Democrats crossed over the party line, gave their votes to Mr. Reagan. Actually Mr. Reagan started his political career as a Democrat. So, he knew Democratic Party's absurdity better than most of us, and took the advantage.

Those Democrats who betrayed the Democratic party got a new name, who are called Reagan Democrats.

Many of the Democrats who made their fortune through Democratic Socialistic government project, gave their soul to Mr. Reagan.

They are all over the country, and many of them are still living in Bloomfield, Michigan.

Easily, and handily he wins the election by beating the incumbent. People were tired of the government, standing on the top of their heads, looking like the shape of reversed pyramid.

As soon as he tootk over the White House, with full support from his party and from the other side, he and his team wasted no time to make the government small and efficient by privatizing and downsizing Government Programs massively. He did not hesitate to push his agenda with full force. He started shutting down unnecessary government program one by one, or as many as he can.

Unfortunately, a lot of people lost their job as a result of his budget cut, who had no idea or knowledge of this political turmoil. Young physicians just got out of medocal school was the first voctims of the killotin which the formerly failed movie actor brought in to thr White House.

This is why. This is what he did, as president. He eliminated the budget for Residency Training Program of entire country with only exception of a few, University hospitals, Military hospitals etc. As a matter of a fact, the government was paying the salery of the resident docters of all the training hospitals. I have no idea how it started, and which was the first one, whether egg or chicken.

But, most likely the hospitals were unwilling or refuse to invest the money for the training of so called "specialist", and, the society needed specialists so bad. So, the government took care of the burden for the people.

Quite naturally, the reality became the government paying the salery of the resident physician, not the hospitals. Mr. Reagan cut off the umbilcal cord, now it becomes the hospital's responsibilty to pay the young doctors. "Pay(?)" Did I say "pay?" Hell, no, no way. They did not pay. Instead, they turned around, and eliminated training program.

As a result of this cut down, just metropolitan Detroit only, thousands of doctors in training lost their job.

Think about. Just imagine how much money the government saved as a result of eliminating this program only. I do not know anyone, or do not have a friend working for Congressional Budget Office. But, the number would be staggering and still piling up even now, and the future. Because the government will never bring back or restart this prgram ever again.

But, it is enormous amount of money just to think about one year only, or next 10, 20 years and so on. The budget saves continues now and forever. Multiply the number of the residents who lost thrir jobs times their salaries, times 10, 20, 30 years, I get headaches.

Only the few of the training hospitals, who can afford to pay the residents, was able to keep and maintain the resident training. They survived, and still produce Specialists for the society.

The government says, "If you can afford it, you can keep it. But, if you cannot, too bad, we are not the answer of your problem anymore."

Now, does it sound familiar? "the smell of capitalism?"

This was just only the beginning.

So many of government programs disappeared from our sight for good, and people loved it. Why? Mr. Reagan turned around our economy by sacrificing the few.

States, and cities copied the same. Even Democratic governors and mayors followed the same.

Downsizing, and priviatizing becme the bible of governing.

Majority of the people were the beneficiary of Mr. Reagan's policy.

By the way, who was the one single person who got the most benefit from the economic turn around Mr. Reagan. It was, surprise, Mr. Bill Clinton. And you know the rest of the story.

Mr. Reagan will be remembered and respected by many including myself, as a highly successful president, who turned around our and world economy from the bottom of the recession to the booming prosperity without the help of any war.

Can you imagine as a person who failed in marriage, and in his profession, but as a president, he became one of the top 3 most respected president in America's history. Definitely top 5, if not top 3.

Then the question is: What has anything to do with me and Mr. Reagan?

Like anybody else, I was affected by his policy indirectly. By the way, tell me if there is anyone who had no impact whatsoever by the sudden drastic change of governing style?

The realty was: When I became second year resident in Internal Medicine, half of my colleague were gone. By the time I became third year resident, more than half of the remaining half were gone. In fact, only a few left. But, you are lucky, if you are one of the few.

Just imagine in the Internal Medicine department, ususlly 10 third year residents were in charge of handling the entire hospital's inpatient and outpatient workload.

All of a sudden, a few left, and workloads were the same or increased. Not to mention about day time work, but as far as night calls, when you become third year residents, you take 3 or 4 times a month in a usual scenario. But, the workload remained the same or worse, because number of my colleagues went down to more than a quarter or worse.

America is such a huge country that it takes a long time for the people to feel the difference if or when Washington changes any law. By the time the general public feel the difference, those who made the changes, those who are responsible, are long gone.

Whether you are are going to be one of the victims or the beneficiaries, you never know what will happen to you unless you are Washington insiders or you are the ones who are making the changes.

So, almost 3 to 4 years of training, number of night calls did not change for me. And, artificial insomnias, caused by against my will, which I did not asked for it, set in me permanently.

But, again, I do not hate Mr. Reagan. As I mentioned earlier, I like him. Further more, I respect him. Because I know that he made all the changes not for himself, but he did it for the benefit of everybody, everyone including my self, and even for Mr. Bill Clinton.

He did it for me, not for himself.

When a politician does something for himself or few of previleged ones, we the people suffer dearly. When a politician does something for the people, we the people get the benefit eventually.

The changes are coming to Health Insurance Industry. The concept of HMO(Health Maintainance Organization) comes in to play big role. I have to say huge role.

Insurance company hires a few doctors and nurses, and they decide whether not to pay or how much the health insurance is going to pay the hospitals and the doctors based on the diagnosis.

Even how long a patient can have in-patient care already determined by those few people. And, the doctors have to discharge in a certain time, instead of necessity.

Everything is dictated by the insurance, even what kind of medicines the doctor can prescribe or not. The doctor has to choose among those medicines that the insurance company pre-selected. Government passed the law which allows the insurance company to come up with taylor-made coverage based on the diagnosis rather than the patient's condition. The doctor or the hospital cannot keep the patient longer than the insurance dictates.

So, when I graduated residency program, and became a staff of Doctor's Group. The environment of medical practice changed drastically. Some days, I have to spend more time arguing insurance companny on the phone, rather than taking care of my sick patients.

After 4 years of practicing in private sector, struggling with health insurance, I decided to move to something or somewhere else, choosing to join the hospital belongs to Department of Correction, State of Michigan.

On one afternoon, on lunch break, my partner said," Hey, do you want to go to Jackson?"

About 40 minutes west of Ann Arbor, in Jackson, Michigan, the biggest walled correctional facility in America is located. The biggest walled correctional facility in America means the biggest in the entire world.

They are housing more than 20 thousand of inmates, and more than 7 thousand correctional officers.

In that facility, there is a small hospital, called Dwayne L Waters Hospital.

It has inpatient bed of 100, Emergency Room, Operation Rooms, Lab, Radiology dept as well. Surgeons, Internist, Psychiatrists, and Dentist, an so on. More than 50 doctors wer working in the Hospital. So, all the sick patiients including terminally ill, come to DLW Hospital receive proper care by the doctor like me, untill they go out healthy, or they pass away.

I went to the hospital, was interviewed by the Medical Director, whose name, by the way, was Dr. Silas Norman, whose sister happened to be Jesse Norman, world famous classic opera singer. He, himself, was also excellent classic baritone singer.

At the end of the interview, he tolld me that, once I chose to work at the hospital, in case I decided to quit the next day due to whatever the reason it might be, come to his office exactly one year later and submit the letter of the resignation. He demanded and I promised to do that.

Bacause he already knew that I have heard all the scary things about inside the wall.

But, somehow, immediately I began to like to work for the prisoners, no the imnates. They were like any other human being, as I treat them, and respect them, they respected me, and treated me like any other human being.

So, I continued to work and treated sick people in the facilty. One year, 2,3,4,5, ten, almost 20 years I work for the people inside of the wall.

Professionally, those years were the best time of my entire life. Certainly, it was Golden days of my life.

It was one of those days. I forgot the date very soon, but you will find out why I remember the exact date if, or when you finish reading this chapter.

It was March 27th, 1992, at lunch.

After spending busy morning as usual, I was enjoying my lunch with other staffs, correction officers, Nurses, and secretaries in a small cafeteria on the first floor.

All of a sudden, I felt a sharp pain on the side of my rib cage. The nurse sitting next to me pinched or poked me without mercy. I do not remember how she did it, with the fork, or her long finger nail.

She was pointing her finger at the correction officer, bending his neck and grabbing his neck with his both hands. I could not see his face, but could see his ear lobes whose color already turned almost black. Though he was a caucacian man. As it turned out, he was a bit older than I am, but much bigger than I am.

Immediately, I recognized the situation. "This is it!"

No time to think. No time to be panic.

Suddenly, no sound, or no noise. There was nobody around. Just him and me.

I found mysely standing behind him. Then I helped him to stand up. No, I put him up. His body had no bone oj joints, and he was very heavy. He was a bit taller than I am. I am 5'10" or 11" tall, he was a bit over 6 feet. But, he was a lot heavier than I am.

He had beard and mustash, and looks like big Santa.

I tried to put my arms around him. It was not easy. Due to his weight, the gravity, the earth is pulling him down constantly, and I had to keep him straight up to apply Heimlich manuever.

At last, the first abdominal thrust.

I thought I did it real hard. But, there was no response.

Here comes the second attempt.

I used all of my reserved muscle strength since I was born. But, I was holding a heavy body with no breathing ready to go where he came from.

So, I had to do it again, the third abdominal thrust. Just before the third trial, only a split second, exactly half of a second, like a lightening, or an electric current, something pass through my brain.

If I put in writing, it is as following;

"If he does not wake up after the third trial, if there is no response, that's the end."

Two things went through my mind. It was a prayer or something.

First, It was directed to God, who was watching from the time it happened. It was almost like half pray, and half threatening Him, whoever He is. "Please save this person. If not, he is going to die now. Then, You are responsible! Not me." Actually, I was begging Him. I was desperate.

Second, If he dies now, what kind of doctor I am going to be in front of all these people. I became a physician to save people's life. I spent all the money, time and energy to be the one who saves people's life. I'm going to be a failure, and all the efforts will be wasted, and gone down the drain."

To tell you the truth, It did not last more than half of one second.

"Boom!!!!" the third attmpt.

I felt his weight became a little bit lighter. I put his body on the foor, and lie down next to him, and look at his face. It seem like human color, living human color. I checked his pulse, and respiration. He had pulse and was breathing. A few minutes later he opened his eyes, and tried to sit up.

And then, 2 or 3 month passed.

On one morning, there was a message that Administrator was looking for me. I went to see him in the afternoon. He said the Warden is the one who wants to see me. He had no idea why.

Next morning, I went to the Warden's office. His office was located in the other building.

As soon as I showed up, he jumped up from his big chair, and offered his big hand with a big smile.

And, he said, "Thank you very much for saving my officer."

He called his secretary to bring Employee of the Month award, and an envelope with some cash. I do not remember how much it was, but enough to have pizzas for lunches with my staffs. There was another page of statement explaining what happened.

"How did you know?" I asked. He said, "I know everything what's happening here."

And then, he said no doctor has ever been given this award in the history of the Michigan's Correction Department. Probably, it is not going to happen in the future either, he said.

Few days later, I met the officer at the same place. And asked him what happened.

At the lunch table, he was about to finish his lunch. He was eating the dessert. A small piece of coocky went into airpipe suddenly, and unexpectedly.

He tried desperately to bring it up on his own, so that he would not ruin other one's lunch. Instead of coming out, the small piece went down further, and he passed out.

He said he did not remember how long he was out, but suddenly saw bright sunlight in his eyes.

Then, he went back to his post. But, he could not continue his duty because of splitting headaches.

He went to his superior and asked his permission to leave early, who asked the reason. Because he rarely left his post early, something never happened before. He told his superior what happened at the lunch table.

The story went up and up through the commanding channel, finally to the warden's office.

But, after 3,4 months later, strange thing started happening, and continued on and on to my body, to be exact, on my shoulder, on my right shoulder.

Initially, it happened only at night, excruciating pain on my right shoulder, waking me up at night, once, twice, then becomes many times.

Then, it occurs during the day.

What is going on? What happened?

The pain gets worse and worse and becomes unbearable.

Finally, I had to go. I had to go to the hospital to find the reason. Hoping it is not something bad.

The doctor ordered XRay of my shoulder.

He came to me with X-Rays, also with interesting looking, and said, "You have separation of right shoulder. Can you think of any reason why? Have you injured your right shoulder lately?"

My Immediate response was "no." The doctor gave me pain medicine, told me to come back if the pain does not go away, I might need surgery if the pain gets worse.

On the way home in the car, out of nowhere, lightening hits me.

"Oh, yes! I did something!" Something called Heimlich manuever.

I remembered what I have done to my shoulder. Most likely I pulled apart my sholder during one of those abdominal thrusts. That's when something happened.

At the same time when I was doing the third attempt, I also remembered that I threatened Someone upstairs, who might have done something to my shoulder.

This nasty pain lasted for more than several years.

Then, it disappeared without telling me. One day it was gone. Even though the pain is gone, the evidence is still there. Separation of my right shoulder still stays with me even now.

By the way, At the beginning of this chapter, I mentioned about which side I choose between American Red Cross, and Heimlich manuever.

As you might have recognized already, I am on the side of Dr. Heimlich.

The reason is;

In a situation of desperation, when life and death is on the line, why are you wasting the time while blowing the victim's back, and then go to the next step, which is Heimlich manuever.

Don't waste any time or thinking, just go to the one that works, which both sides does not disfute.

That's what I did.

Opportunity is bald on the back. You can grab it only on the front. If you miss the front, no way you can grab the opportunity from behind. Once you miss it, there is no such thing called second chance. when we are dealing with human life, your life and my life.

Chapter XVIII

Las Vegas, the Sin City?

Why? Why, the sin city?

People living in Las Vegas are sinners? Just because they are living in Las Vegas?

Or, people who went to Las Vegas for a nice vacation, or for business, become sinners when they come back home?

Certainly not.

Actually, the citizens of Las Vegas like to call their city Entertainment Capital of the World.

But, depending on what you do in Las Vegas with your hard earn money, Vegas bocomes Sin City or Entertainment Capital.

Living in Ann Arbor, Michigan.

I like to go to Las Vas in winter. Winter only. Only in winter. You can stay in Michigan the rest of the year. If you enjoy winter weather, and winter sports, you do not need to go anywhere else. Just stay in Michigan.

I do agree that the weather in winter season in nothern states is really cold, particularly cruel in nothern parts of states like

Michigan, Minnesota, Wisconsin, New York, etc, not to mention Canada.

So, I'm one of the many who needs to go warm place in winter, once or twice, the more the better.

Quite naturally, Las Vegas became one of my favorite destination I like to go in winter time.

It became a lot better, and warmer in winter in Michigan due to global warming compared to 10, 20, 30 or 40 years ago.

But, by the time December comes, cold gets colder, I have to go somewhere, somewhere I can relax. I guess I'm one of those who suffers from a condition called "cabin fever."

Generally my favorite destination is Florida, or Cancun, Mexico in January when I need to melt down my frozen mind, and Las Vegas in February when I need a little bit of entertainment along with warm weather.

When March is here, winter is gone in Michigan.

Now, I'm about to talk about Las Vegas.

But, to tell you the truth, although it is good place to have a fun, Vegas is not a good place to live. I have friends who moved to Las Vegas after retiring. But, I have no intention to move to Vegas after my retirement.

As usual, bad news first.

Not a good place to live? Two things comes into my mind, weather and gambling. Maybe, in terms of winter weather, Vegas has one of the best. However, the rest of the year, remember where Vegas is locsted. Next to Mojabee desert and right next to Death Valley.

And, the entire city is filled with casinos.

Next, the good news!

Can you think of any city better than Vegas in terms of entertainment.

Excellent scenery, good sightseeing, so many places to go, so many things to do, so many good places to eat, etc.

It is Entertainment Capital of the World. I agre 100%.

Let's talk about gambling, ie casinos.

Recently, in USA, casinos popped up everywhere, big city or small city, it doesn't matter. It is worrisome reality, but instesd of worrying, it's time to find solution on our own. In the past, it was watching fire across the street, or across the river, now it became fire on my shoes.

In the past, in order to go to casino, we have to go to Las Vegas, or Atlantic City, which means we have go there by air.

Now, if we want to go to casino, we can drive less than an hour on any direction.

Why? By whom?

First, by whom? By politician is the answer.

Why? In American politics, there is one thing politician should never say, even while in his sleep. It is tax. Never talk about increasing tax, no matter how good the intention may be.

No matter how bad the economy may be, if he mentions about tax hike to solve the problem, the moment he or she says, he or she is dead politically.

Even if he or she got elected, never talk about increasing taxes.

During campaign for the first term, wherever he may go, single term president, father Bush said to the audience, pointing his lips "Read my lips. No new taxes." But, he increased tax as soon as he became the president. That was his fatal mistake for his second term election.

So, we don't know whose idea it was, where it came from.

Casino became the solution.

By taking advantage of gambling "gene" that we all have, Billionares, not millionares, will collect money with ease from average person like you or me. And, politicians collect tax from casino. They don't have to increase tax. It is just a matter of time for average Joe to go bankrupt.

As a result, casinos are popping up everywhere. Here in Ann Arbor, it takes only 30 or 40 minutes to go to downtown Detroit, where 3 big casinos are enjoying booming business. From Detroit to Winsor, Canada, taking only 10 minutes or so, we can reach one of the biggest casino in Canada.

From Ann Arbor to Toledo, Ohio, taking 30 to 40 minutes, there is another huge casino.

From Ann Arbor, to the West, about one hour distance, another casino is waiting for average Joe. Open 24 hours, day and night, they are waiting. Who cares whether he goes bankrupt or not. No one cares.

Something that we did not witness before.

It is becoming social issues. No, it became social issue already.

Gun violence, drug addiction, alcoholism, and gambling.

I worry about the future of America. I worry about my future, and my future generations an so on.

Among addictions, we can think about following 5. Alcohol, Nicotine, drug addiction, then food, and gambling addiction.

I'm going to talk about why we shouldn't go Vegas first, then why we should go next.

Before gambling, let's talk about alcoholism.

Generally, there are 3 different group of people.

First, people born with sufficient amount of gene, ie alcoholc gene. So, no matter how much, what kind of alcohol he or she may drink, it doesn't bother him or her. We call them Supermen. But, at end, ultimately, the person ruins not only his body, but also his mind, and ruins not only himself, but also his innocent family.

Second, people born with no or almost no gene, so that his face turns red even with smell of alcohol.

Third, someone in the middle, more than second group, but a lot less than the first. So, that if this person happened to be surrounded by first group, quite naturally, he becomes alcoholic. If, surrounded by second group of people, he remains and belongs to second group.

Definition of alcoholism has nothing to do with the amount of alcohol. So, the definition is as follows,: "any drinking alcohol that results in problem." If drinking alcohol causes any problem to you, your family, your job, ultimately to the society, you are alcoholic. You have alcohol addiction. If you have problem, the society have problem.

Back to gambling, as in alcoholism,

First, people born with sufficient amount of gambling gene, are living with high probability to get addicted, and once exposed, there is high chance to ruin not only his life, but also his family.

Second, people who are born with no gene or almost no gene, are living without urge to go to casino. This people have no chance or almost no chance to get addicted.

Third, someone who are in the middle, more genes than the second group, a lot less than the first. So, that if this person happened to be surrounded by first group, he remains and belongs to first group. But, this person happened to be surrounded by second group, he will belong, and remain second group.

I sincerely hope and pray for the people in third group and second group as well.

But, there is only one exception.

You are retired, all the retirement plans are in place. You are old and accomplished. Why not! Give all your assets to your next generation already. And then, with your leftover, enjoy your life, whichever way you choose. Gambling is good for the prevention of dementia. But, if you have dementia, hopely you forgot about gambling as well.

Followings are the reasons why we shouldn't gambling.

One, There is no chance. No probabability. Why do you start a war when you know you are going to lose.

Because it is fun? What kind of fun is that? Are you having fun to lose your hard earn money. Nonsense!

We have no chance with table game. The longer you sit there, for sure the less your chance will be. You have to decide whether to stay or fold before the dealer. What a disadvantage it is! What a nonsense.

Statistically, the chance to lose or win is 49% to 51%, it's pretty high, but do not be fooled by the nunbers.

And, in slot machine, it is worse, much worse than table game.

A personal story heard from a taxi driver. More than 10 years, he worked hard day and night as a dealer to save enough money to own and run a small buisiness. When he said to hinself that the time has come, he decided to go to the casino where he used to work as a customer, not as a dealer just for one day, only one day only.

That one day became 2 days, then 3 days and so on. All his money's gone, and he could not leave Vegas, and became a taxi driver.

Two, again we, average Joe, lose again. This time, it is psychological warfafe. Geniuses in math and psychology graduated from Ivy League, Big 10, Pac 10 are working for casinos behind the curtain. We, average Joes, are no match for those geniuses. Give up to win in casino against these people, geniuses. You, and I are no match.

3 Nos in casino

No window to look outside. We cannot see outside, cannot see reality. No chance to other people, average gambler like myself. No chance to see reality outside.

No mirrors around you. Except when you are in the rest rooms. You cannot see your face while gambling. You cannot see your face, the face of loser's.

No clocks on the wall. Unless you have your own watch. You cannot tell or see whether the sun is out, or the moon is out.

So, once you step in the casino, you lose the concept time, and numbers and so on.

Especially, you lose the concept of money. The value of the money disappears. Someone, who goes to grocery stores or department stores, looking for items one dollar cheaper.

All of s sudden, he or she throws away 100 dollar bill on the table like one dollar bill.

In the whole USA, no one can smoke inside of any of public places, but there is only one exception, that is casinos. You can smoke in casinos in USA, but not in Canada.

When I go to Vegas, I see someone that I know who moved to Vegas from Michigan.

They say Vegas is so good that they highly, and highly recommend anybody to move to Vegas after retiring. They say it was the best decision that they have ever made to move to Vegas.

But, they never fail to mention at the end, "Vegas will be your dream come true, only, only if you have the will power to stay away from casinos."

So, throw away your greed, and open the window of your mind, then something good will fly into your mind.

Now, the reason we have to go to Vegas.

For your own information, among the lists of places that people want to go on winter vacation.

Public poll shows:

#1, Las Vegas

#2, Cancun, Mexico

#3, Orlando, Florida, where Disney World is located.

First,

Even though it is part of the reason why I do not recommend to move after retiring due to hot summer weather, where can you find a better place for entertainment in the world than Vegas for winter vacation.

I have never been to Las Vegas in summer time so far. So, I cannot comment about summer weather in Vegas, again, death valley is only 2 hours away from Vegas. That's all I can say.

Anyway, if you go to Vegas in winter, the weather feels like late autumn. When the sun is out, it is warm. But, when the sun goes down, it is quite chilly. That is all for the weather

Second,

To attract the casino customers, the other expenses are relatively cheaper than you think. Prices of hotel, airplane, food, etc. There are many excellent shows, performances every where.

Talking about food, the city has top 10 buffet reatraunt in the whole USA. When we say the city is the Entertainment Capital of the World, it also include entertaining our taste buds in our body.

Third,

You can go to the Grand Cannyon. And, Hoover Dam.

One is God made, the other is man made. How magnificent these two are.

I'm not going to describe Grand Cannyon, because it's impossible. It is as simple as that. It is impossible. You have to see it to believe it.

People are coming all over the world. Tourists are coming to Las Vegas to see Grand Cannuon.

Fourth,

If you drive to the direction of Utah state, about 2 and half hours, you will meet Zion Cannyon National Park, about 4 hours, Bryce Cannyon National park.

Again, I'm not going to describe about how magnificent they are.

But, especially, when you go to Zion National Park, you don't want to come home.

You want to stay there for good.

Fifth,

There are many, good golf courses around the city. Golf is excellent tool to stay away from gambling.

Sixth,

Excellent shows, performances in the evening.

Seventh,

2 hours from Vegas. You can visit Death Valley. There is hot spring, I was told.

If you are involved in all of these activities, you do not have much time to sit on the gambling table. Make yourself busy, and stay away from casino. Spend more time outside.

Believe it or not.

Long, Long time ago, there was a very rich man. When he was about to die, he pray to God that he can carry his hard earn fortune all his life. His prayer was so intense, God could not refuse.

He got the permission from God.

With all his money, he bought gold, thinking that only gold is accepted in the Heaven. Finalliy, when he died, he entered the gate of the Heaven, with his gold on his back, sweating all over his body.

Upon his arrival, people in the heaven were whispering, "We have gold everywhere here. Why he has to sweat for gold." Indeed, he saw gold everywhere in the Heaven. Buildings, streets, everywhere he saw gold. And, everything was free. We do not need money in heaven.

When we go to the Heaven, leave everything behind, and then go with empty handed.

At the moment we came to this world; we are screaming as hard as we can, as if somebody beat us up real bad. We make our fist as hard as we can, as if we have something precious in our hands, although we had nothing in our hands, or as if we are a boxer ready to fight,

But, when we are ready to go back to where we came from:

We close our eyes softly, so that we can open our eyes any time to see God any moment. We keep our hands empty, so that we can grab His Hands strongly with our two hands. If we are holding something already in our hands, how can we grab His Hands? Humbly we put our hands in the front so that we can grab His Hands real quick, rather than in the back, then how can He grab our hands if we are hiding our hands on the back.

And, two ears are wide open, our mouth shut, so we are ready to hear any thing but we are done talking.

This is the way we are, when we go back where we came from.

Chapter XIX

Conclusion

As a matter of fact, the main subject of this book is health.

When I'm talking about health related subjects, I always put the conclusion, ie the solution, and the answer at the end of the each chapter.

Again, the solution for the good health is Exercise. Exercise, exercise, and exercise. And, work out, work out, and work out.

It does not matter how old you are. It doesnot matter whether you are female or male.

Even if you are paralyzed on a certain part of your body, you have to exercise those part of your body that you can move.

Exercise is essentials, not luxuary. Exercise is something that you have to do. It is not something that you do if you can, or something you do not do if you cannot.

You do not have to do Stair Exercise which I recommend the most. You do not have to do it, only because I recommend.

It does not matter, as long as it fits the definition of the exercise.

If it fits for your particular condition, your ability, or you can develop a certain exercise fitting just for you, then that is the best exercise for you.

If you have your kind of exercise already, I recommend you to continue your exercise, and add one of those that I recommend.

It does not matter if the methods are different, as long as we reach the same goal. It is important to arrive at the same finish line, and cut the tape with our big chest, and strong, muscular lower extermities.

The finish line of each exercise is to give our body the gift of Respiratory Alkalosis + Endorphin.

We, humans, are are unique, and mysterious creature, that we have to do exercise all the time. We even did exercise before we were born. Sometimes, we kicked mamas' side so hard that mama has to wake up in the middle of the night. We were swimming before we were born.

If you look at newborn babies, they exercise all the time except when they are sleeping.

We like to watch those atheletes whom we like. When my favorite Tigers hits a home run, I feel like I did it. Almost I confuse myself with the athlete I like.

That's how much we like to exercise.

So, I put all the solutions together in one sentence again;

The path to the good health should be the combination of proper exercise, drinking water wisely, and sleep well.

And then, keep your oral hygiene decent, while you take Aspirin and Zantac, aka Acid Reducer once a day.

If I make a formula combining all above;

Good health = (Good Exercise) + (Drink wisely) + (Sleep well) on the top of

(Good oral hygiene) + (one ASA a day) + (one Acid Reducer aka Zantac)

Work hard what you do every day, and save enough money for your hobby, hopefully it's travelling.

And, enjoy travelling. I recommend travelling.

Travelling overseas, just think about it, it makes me get excited.

I had 3 places to recommend, maybe 4.

Rome, Alaska, Barcellona, and Egypt.

Once is not enough, twice is not enough, and so on. Like an old friend, who grew up together, do not need to talk, just looking at each other is more than enough. This meeting could be the last, but still promising each other to meet again like an old friend.

First, easy one.

Barcellona, Spain.

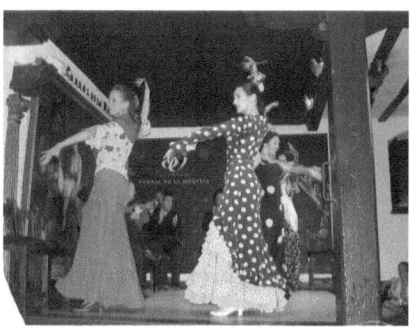
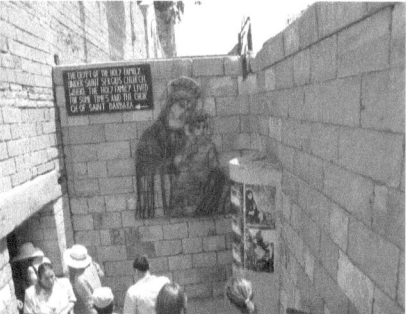

I recommend group tour. This is not a small country located east end of Europe, along with Portugal.

When you go to Spain, always include Madrid and Barcellona. If you are a catholic, make sure to visit Mont Serrat an hour from Barcellona. Also make sure you have enough time to meet Black Madonna.

Next, Rome

It is the best place to travel alone or with just few good friends, or two couples, after you had a chance or two to get familiaririze, or get to know each other, you and Rome. I have seen many solitary traveller.

If you study or research about history of Italy, then you will learn a lot more after each travel, that will make you want to go Rome over, and over again.

In fact, it is very safe place to travel Europe, especially Rome, Italy. You do not have to worry about safety.

When you go to Rome alone or with a few, utilize public transportation, especially bus. Because you can see outside in the bus.

Another thing that you must not forget is hotel close to "Terminale."

When you go to Rome, include another place or city of different variety, such as Milano, Venice, Florence, Santa Lucia, etc.

Alaska.

I recommend solo travelling, or with a few from the first trip. Unlike any other travelling, you need peace and quiet. Two couple would be ideal.

Sometimes, you have to choose in a group, or entire famly travelling together like cruise.

Other than special occasions, if you want to mix with nature and become one, I highly recommend Alaska travel you alone or just a few.

Alaska is closest from the continent of US among those places I recommend.

Go to Anchorage first, and rent a car, a SUV, a miniVan, or a RV, etc at the airport, whatever you want, and go wherever you want. As far as I know Alaska Airport is the only one that you can rent a RV.

You must include Denali in Alaska trip. I mean Denali National Park.

As you studied before you start, drive wherever as GPS tells you to go.

Egypt, last, but not the least.

You have to travel in a group from the beginning. You have to consider your safety, also.

Like any other travel, you have to study real hard about the history of ancient Egypt if you want to make the most out of this particular travel.

You have to choose a travel package which includes Nile River Cruise, and Abu Simbel and spend at least 2 weeks in Egypt.

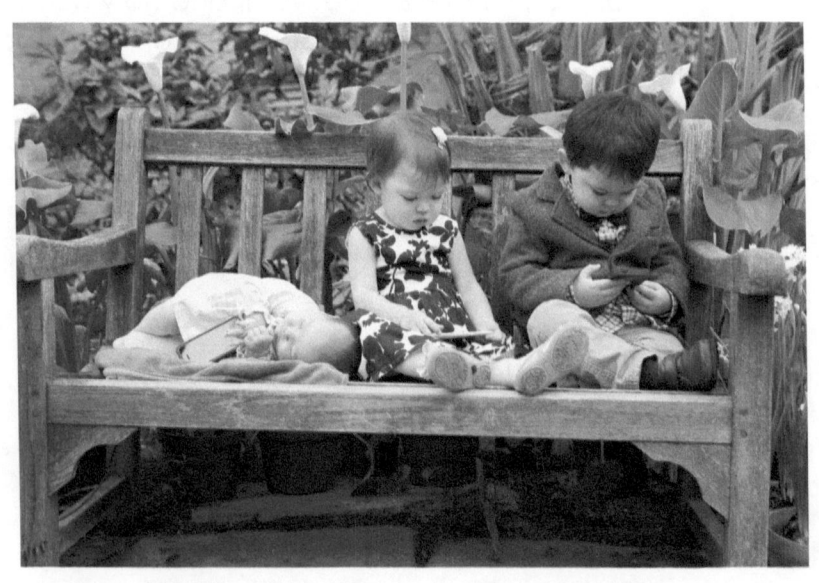